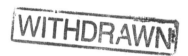

OXFORD MEDICAL PUBLICATIONS

Paediatric Day Case Surgery

Paediatric Day Case Surgery

Edited by

N. S. Morton

Consultant in Paediatric Anaesthesia and Intensive Care
Royal Hospital for Sick Children
Glasgow

and

P. A. M. Raine

Consultant in Paediatric Surgery
Royal Hospital for Sick Children
Glasgow
Barclay Lecturer in Paediatric Surgery
University of Glasgow

Oxford   New York   Tokyo
OXFORD UNIVERSITY PRESS
1994

Oxford University Press, Walton Street, Oxford OX2 6DP

Oxford New York Toronto
Delhi Bombay Calcutta Madras Karachi
Kuala Lumpur Singapore Hong Kong Tokyo
Nairobi Dar es Salaam Cape Town
Melbourne Auckland Madrid
and associated companies in
Berlin Ibadan

Oxford is a trade mark of Oxford University Press

Published in the United States
by Oxford University Press Inc., New York

© *N. S. Morton, P. A. M. Raine, and the contributors listed on p. xi, 1994*

A catalogue record for this book is available from the British Library

Library of Congress Cataloging in Publication Data
(Data available upon request)

ISBN 0 19 262256 0

Typeset by Advance Typesetting Ltd, Oxfordshire
Printed in Hong Kong

Foreword

by P. Morris

Consultant Paediatric Anaesthetist, Immediate Past President,
Association of Paediatric Anaesthetists of Great Britain and Ireland

Recent years have seen pressure from many sources to increase day surgery. The advantages of this important element of surgical care, not purely for economic reasons, have now been generally accepted. With regard to surgery in childhood the advantages are very clear, facilitating the concept of parental participation in care, while minimizing the stress of the child's hospital admission and disruption to the family. However, as with the delivery of other aspects of health care to children, their special needs and those of their parents must be recognized and provided for.

Organization and management of the day unit, with concise selection criteria for anaesthesia and surgery incorporating a team approach, is all important. Furthermore, the availability of clear and comprehensive written information for parents is essential and cannot be over-emphasized.

Paediatric day surgery has its origins in Glasgow and it is fitting that those providing this service in that city today have collaborated to produce this book. The many contributors under the expert guidance of the editors, Dr N. S. Morton and Mr P. A. M. Raine, have drawn on their extensive personal experience to produce a 'state of the art' account of all aspects of the subject, commendable for its clarity. Although the book relies heavily on practice in one large British children's centre, the delivery of paediatric day surgery is bound to be modified and adapted to the particular environment in which it is practised. Whether this is in a specialist or district general hospital in the UK, or overseas, the principles of day care remain the same. This book contains up-to-date information and sound practical clinical advice for those interested in day case surgery in children. I recommend this text as a reliable, readable account of current practice.

Preface

This book aims to bring together in a single text the essential principles underlying modern paediatric day case anaesthesia and surgery. Careful patient selection is therefore paramount. Detailed inclusion and exclusion criteria are discussed and tabulated. The techniques of anaesthesia, analgesia, and surgery are described and illustrated in colour. Trainees in surgery, anaesthesia, and nursing will find the text useful with up-to-date references for further reading. Established consultants in district hospitals (where much paediatric surgery is still carried out), will find guidance as to which children are suitable for day care and how facilities may be adapted to carry this out safely.

With the continuing expansion of day surgery, it is vital that proper community follow-up at home is organized. General practitioners and their staff will find this book useful in explaining the techniques currently used.

Practice varies throughout this country, Europe, North America, and Australia. The motivation behind day care is often financial, but it is important that considerations of safety predominate. Clinicians must resist pressure from management teams to extend day care if adequate safeguards cannot be provided. This applies in all fields of medicine but particularly to the care of children after surgery.

Although paediatric day care anaesthesia and surgery demands high standards of skill from experienced staff, the need for teaching and training of junior staff must be taken into account in the planning and running of a day surgery programme.

There is no doubt that children benefit more than most from day care, where minimal separation from parents, home, environment, and school will reduce the psychological upset of having an operation. With good preparation before surgery and careful follow-up care afterwards, paediatric day case anaesthesia and surgery is safe and is preferred by children, parents, and staff.

Royal Hospital for Sick Children, N.S.M.
Glasgow P.A.M.R.
March 1994

Contents

x   Contents

Contributors

D. S. Arthur, M.B.Ch.B., F.R.C.A., Consultant in Paediatric Anaesthesia; Clinical Director of Anaesthesia, Theatres and Intensive Care, RHSC, Glasgow; Honorary Clinical Senior Lecturer, University of Glasgow

D. Attwood, B.D.S., M.P.H., Ph.D., Consultant in Dentistry, RHSC, Glasgow; Honorary Clinical Lecturer in Child Dental Health, University of Glasgow

A. A. F. Azmy, M.B.Ch.B., D.S., F.R.C.S.(Lon.,Glas.), Consultant in Paediatric Surgery, RHSC, Glasgow; Honorary Clinical Senior Lecturer, University of Glasgow

G. C. Bennet, B.Sc., M.B.Ch.B., F.R.C.S., Consultant in Orthopaedic Surgery, RHSC, Glasgow; Honorary Clinical Senior Lecturer, University of Glasgow

C. J. Best, M.B.B.S., F.R.C.A., Consultant in Paediatric Anaesthesia, RHSC, Glasgow

J. G. Boorman, B.Sc., M.B.Ch.B., F.R.C.S.(Eng.), Consultant in Plastic Surgery, East Grinstead (formerly RHSC, Glasgow)

J. Dudgeon, M.B.Ch.B., F.R.C.S.(Glas.,Eng.), D.O., F.C.Oph., Consultant in Ophthalmology, RHSC, Glasgow; Honorary Clinical Senior Lecturer, University of Glasgow

D. J. M. Fretwell, R.S.C.N., Formerly Sister in Charge, Day Surgery Unit, RHSC, Glasgow

A. H. B. Fyfe, M.B.Ch.B., F.R.C.S.(Glas.), Consultant in Paediatric Surgery, RHSC, Glasgow; Honorary Clinical Senior Lecturer, University of Glasgow

N. K. Geddes, M.B.Ch.B., F.R.C.S.(Glas.), Consultant in Otorhinolaryngology, RHSC, Glasgow; Honorary Clinical Senior Lecturer, University of Glasgow

L. R. McNicol, M.B.Ch.B., F.R.C.A., Consultant in Paediatric Anaesthesia, RHSC, Glasgow

1 A historical perspective

D. S. Arthur and N. S. Morton

The first use of general anaesthesia for day case surgery was on 30 March 1842 when Crawford Long of Jefferson, Georgia excised a small tumour from the neck of a friend. This was not only the first day case under general anaesthesia, but the first case of surgical anaesthesia recorded. Later William Morton introduced ether anaesthesia at the Massachusetts General Hospital on 16 October 1846. The concept rapidly crossed the Atlantic and was introduced to the old world in Dumfries and Galloway Infirmary on 19 December 1846. Prior to the introduction of general anaesthesia, surgery was relatively uncommon even in large teaching hospitals in the UK, 120 operations being carried out per year in the Glasgow Royal Infirmary (Watt 1961). General anaesthesia changed this and also allowed day case surgery to be carried out, particularly for dental extractions. An early photograph of Joseph Clover using his chloroform inhaler demonstrates its use in a day patient (Fig. 1.1). Unfortunately the first reported death due to chloroform in the UK also occurred in a day case undergoing

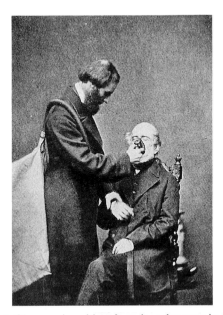

Fig. 1.1   Joseph Clover using chloroform in a day case in 1862. (From the original photograph, presented by his daughter, Miss Mary Clover, to the Nuffield Department of Anaesthetics, Oxford)

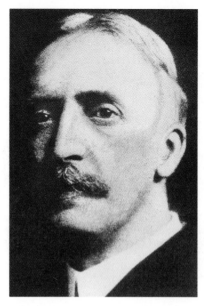

Fig. 1.2 J. H. Nicoll (1864–1921)

surgery for removal of a toe-nail in January 1848. Chloroform continued to be popular for paediatric anaesthesia in particular and was most likely the anaesthesia used for patients operated on by James Nicoll (Fig. 1.2).

Nicoll presented his experience of paediatric day cases operated on in the Sick Children's Hospital Dispensary in Glasgow (Figs 1.3, 1.4) in the British Medical Journal of 18 September 1909 (Nicoll 1909). He reported a series of 9000 procedures carried out over the ten years from 1899 to 1908; of these he himself performed 7392. At a meeting in Belfast, Nicoll expounded his reasons for operating on children as day cases. The five conclusions he reached then are as pertinent today.

Nicoll noted firstly that 'much surgery done in hospital was a waste of resources' and that the cost of day case surgery was a tenth of that for the in-patient equivalent.

He advocated careful selection of cases although his choice might be questioned today. Selection will be discussed in the next chapter. His second observation was that bed rest following surgery although 'a pretty idea' was virtually impossible to achieve in infants and children to such an extent that some had to be splinted to the bed to maintain the so called benefits of bed rest. Nicoll also noted that unfortunately 'children in a ward are not infrequently noisy and malodorous'. The main idea of admission was 'the supposed benefit of trained nursing' but with a mother of average intelligence the child fared better at home

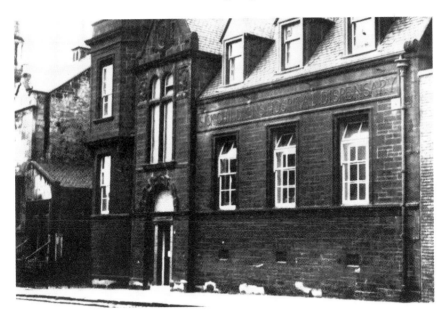

Fig. 1.3 The Sick Children's Hospital Dispensary, West Graham Street, Glasgow

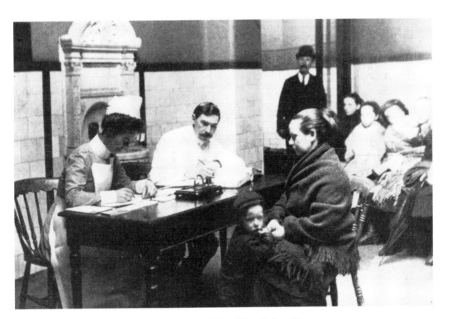

Fig. 1.4 Professor Nicoll's clinic, Glasgow

than in hospital. This was aided by his far-sighted approach in employing nursing sisters who visited the child on his return home to assist the mother with any problems that should occur. This concept is very strongly advised today in any well organized day case department.

A further benefit for the child remaining with its mother was that of feeding, particularly in the case of the breast-fed infant. Separation of the child from the mother even in the absence of breast-feeding was harmful. This important aspect of paediatric surgery was fostered by Nicoll in a most altruistic way in that he personally provided a house where mother and child could be together, and he proposed that 'no children's hospital could be considered complete if it did not provide accommodation for mothers to stay with their children'.

Nicoll appreciated that the turnover of cases could be more rapid by reducing the time under anaesthesia. Performing almost 1000 operations per year lends some credibility to his argument.

Lastly he extrapolated his experience with children to his adult practice and suggested that they also were kept in bed too long following surgery. It was obvious from the proceedings of the meeting where Nicoll presented his views that he was not alone, and that others in Edinburgh, Belfast, and Liverpool were also carrying out paediatric day case surgery.

Dental surgery continued to be the most frequently performed surgery under general anaesthesia until the last few decades and it was his experience of this type of surgery that encouraged Ralph Waters (1919), who introduced cyclopropane to anaesthesia, to open his downtown anaesthesia clinic where surgeons came with their patients for the operation. In this case economics were again the driving factor.

Reports of the success and benefits of paediatric day case surgery continued to appear sporadically (Lawrie 1964), but it was not until 1967 that the first reports of purpose built day care units at the Hammersmith Hospital appeared (Calman and Martin 1971).

Continuing escalation in the cost of medical care in the United States in particular promoted the establishment of the downtown Surgicentre quite separate from any hospital, the first being built in Phoenix, Arizona in 1970 (Reed and Ford 1976). Other units followed rapidly to such an extent that today justification has to be made to insurance companies in the USA to perform certain types of procedure as in-patients. The success of the purpose built unit at Cambridge, UK has been described by Ogg (1989). The Royal College of Surgeons of England (1985) produced a report extolling the virtues and encouraging the increased use of day case surgery.

More recently the organization Caring for Children in the Health Service has examined the benefits of paediatric day care, from both the economic point of view and more particularly from the point of view of the child and the benefits to him or her in the avoidance of a hospital stay, whether for surgery or medical investigation and treatment.

A report (Thornes 1991) was produced by this multidisciplinary group comprising nurses, paediatricians, surgeons, an anaesthetist, and members of the National Association for the Welfare of Children in Hospital. It presented useful practical advice and these 12 quality standards for all children admitted as day cases:

1. The admission is planned in an integrated way to include pre-admission, day of admission, and post-admission care, and to incorporate the concept of a planned transfer of care to primary and/or community services.
2. The child and parent are offered preparation, both before and during the day of admission.
3. Specific written information is provided to ensure that parents understand their responsibilities throughout the episode.
4. The child is admitted to an area designated for day cases and not mixed with acutely ill in-patients.
5. The child is neither admitted nor treated alongside adults.
6. The child is cared for by identified staff specifically designated to the day case area.
7. Medical, nursing, and all other staff are trained for, and skilled in, work with children and their families, in addition to the expertise needed for day case work.
8. The organization and delivery of patient care are planned specifically for day cases so that every child is likely to be discharged within the day.
9. The building, equipment, and furnishings comply with safety standards for children.
10. The environment is homely and includes areas for play and other activities designed for children and young people.
11. Essential documentation, including communication with primary care and/or community services, is completed before each child goes home so that after-care and follow-up consultations are not delayed.
12. Once care has been transferred to the home, nursing support is provided, at a doctor's request, by nurses trained in the care of sick children.

References

Calman, J. and Martin, P. (1971). Development and practice of an autonomous minor surgery unit in a general hospital. *British Medical Journal*, **iv**, 92.

Lawrie, A. (1964). Operating on children as day cases. *Lancet*, **ii**, 1289.

Nicoll, J. H. (1909). The surgery of infancy. *British Medical Journal*, **ii**, 753–6.

Ogg, T. W. (1989). Establishing a day care unit. In *Day care surgery, anaesthesia and management* (ed. E. G. Bradshaw and H. T. Davenport), pp. 13–24. Edward Arnold, London.

Reed, W. A. and Ford, J. L. (1976). Development of an independent outpatient surgical centre. *International Anaesthesiology Clinics*, 14–130.

Royal College of Surgeons of England. (1985). *Guidelines for day case surgery.* Commission on the Provision of Surgical Services. Royal College of Surgeons of England, London.

Thornes, R. (1991). *Just for the day.* NAWCH Ltd, London.

Waters, R. M. (1919). The downtown anaesthesia clinic. *American Journal of Surgery*, **33**, 71–3.

Watt, O. M. (1961). *Glasgow anaesthetists 1846 to 1946.* University of Glasgow.

2 Facilities for paediatric day case surgery

N. S. Morton

The ideal provision for paediatric day case surgery is in a children's day unit, admitting both surgical and medical cases and other ambulatory patients. This is not always possible but a children's in-patient ward can have an area within it adapted for day treatment which has separate staff, policies, and operational rules. If children have to be admitted to an adult day surgical unit, then separate sessions or separate facilities for children should be established. Whatever the local arrangements, the 12 quality standards noted in Chapter 1 (Thornes 1991) should be followed when designing the environment for paediatric day case surgery, staffing the unit, and organizing and delivering patient care.

The *environment* of the day case unit should be appropriate for children and separated from in-patients. Children need not be confined to bed in the preoperative period and the unit must therefore be equipped to cope with active children. Fitments which are safe and appropriate for children should be used to create a friendly environment. Facilities for parents and a direct dial telephone line are essential. A fully equipped treatment room for procedures such as venepuncture, plaster work, administration of chemotherapy, etc. must be provided. The anaesthetic induction room and operating theatre may be integral to the unit, but this carries with it the problem of the isolated anaesthetic location. If the induction room and operating theatre are part of a suite, they must be appropriately decorated and equipped for children, with separation from adult patients in reception and recovery areas. The design should allow the separation of pre- from postoperative patients. The reception, induction, and recovery areas should be large enough to allow parental involvement with the conscious child.

The *staff*, headed by a director and administrative manager, should include an appropriate skill mix of nursing staff trained in the care of sick children. Play staff and clerical staff are vital for the smooth running of the unit. Surgeons and anaesthetists should be experienced paediatric practitioners and such work should not be delegated to trainees unless they are under the closest personal supervision. The volume of work in different age groups must be adequate to maintain anaesthetic and surgical skills. The operating theatre staff should be trained for day surgery and for work with children and their parents. A trained nurse should be available for parental support.

The *organization and delivery* of patient care must be well planned and co-ordinated from the pre-admission phase to the follow-up phase at home. An advisory group should assist the unit director with planning. Booking arrangements, parental information, and instructions and liaison with community services, must all be well organized and unambiguous. The administrative system should be audited regularly to identify and correct problems, with the views of parents and children playing an important part.

Financial aspects

A customized day case unit is costly to set up, with staff costs a major component (Morton *et al.* 1991). In smaller district hospitals, however, it is possible to show financial savings when the switch is made from in-patient to day case paediatric surgery (Sadler *et al.* 1992). The closure of in-patient beds in larger institutions as a result of starting day case surgery, may save money overall (Ogg 1990). Alternatively, freed in-patient beds may be used for other groups of patients with a consequent reduction in waiting time for in-patient treatment.

The day surgery unit's facilities can be used for patients other than surgical day cases with children attending for investigations, blood sampling, vene-section, chemotherapy etc. In some units the beds are hired out for research purposes to generate income (e.g. at weekends) and this may help the financial viability of the unit (Ogg 1990).

It is important that the operating theatre time is used efficiently. Minimizing cancellations is cost-effective and can be done by telephone canvassing, running a reserve list, improving communication with parents and even preoperative home visiting (Kleinfeldt 1990; Postuma *et al.* 1987). Sessional cancellations due to senior medical staff leave are a problem, but it is possible with good planning to cross cover some of these.

In conclusion, a well designed unit with carefully planned operational policies, equipment, and staff appropriate for children are essential. Patient selection, preparation, and follow-up must be well organized by senior medical and nursing staff. An efficient paediatric day case surgery service is cost-effective and results in a reduction in waiting lists. Patient and parental satisfaction is high and staff enjoy working in this type of unit. Day case surgery is an essential part of modern paediatric care.

References

Kleinfeldt, A. S. (1990). Pre-operative phone calls. Reducing cancellations in paediatric day surgery. *Association of Operating Room Nurses Journal*, **51**, 1559–64.

Morton, N. S., Arthur, D. S., Cattanach, D., Fyfe, A., Best, C. J., and Haynes, K. A. (1991). Day case surgery for children. *Health Bulletin*, **49**, 54–61.

Ogg, T. W. (1990). Day case surgery. *Drug and Therapeutics Bulletin*, **28**, 22–85.

Postuma, R., Ferguson, C. C., Stanwick, R. S., and Horne, J. M. (1987). Paediatric day care surgery : a 30 year hospital experience. *Journal of Paediatric Surgery*, **22**, 304–7.

Sadler, G. P., Richards, H., Watkins, G., and Foster, M. E. (1992). Day case paediatric surgery; the only choice. *Annals of the Royal College of Surgeons of England*, **74**, 130–3.

Thornes, R. (1991). *Just for the day*. NAWCH Ltd, London.

3 Patient selection, assessment, and preoperative preparation

D. S. Arthur, N. S. Morton, and A. H. B. Fyfe

Patient selection and assessment

Many surgical procedures carried out on children are suitable for day care, particularly general surgical, urological, ophthalmological, and ENT procedures (Table 3.1). It is an important decision to select those children who are candidates for day care and those who would be more appropriately treated as in-patients.

A preoperative anaesthetic clinic assists in the preparation and selection of children for day case surgery, but time does not allow most anaesthetists such an opportunity to see the patients before the day of surgery. Guidelines are therefore required for the surgeon in selecting patients seen at the out-patient clinic for in-patient or day care surgery (Table 3.2).

Psychosocial

The financial advantages of day care have been widely reported and, with increasing exhortations to provide value for money in medical care, it is important that patients are not pressurized into inappropriate treatment simply to cut costs.

The advantages of day care for most patients and parents are clear: the absence of parental separation, the requirement to organize the care of other children for one day only, and parental involvement in the patient's care benefit the whole family (Table 3.3).

In spite of these undoubted advantages, many parents may feel unable to care for their child following surgery. The single parent may have difficulty with other children. Those with poor housing, inadequate transport or no telephone, and those who may have to travel long distances to the hospital are often better cared for as in-patients.

The availability of a community nurse to assist the parents in the days following surgery, will reduce the numbers requiring in-patient admission and will increase the confidence of parents in looking after their children.

Table 3.1 Range of procedures carried out as day cases in children

General surgery
Herniotomy (inguinal, femoral, epigastric, umbilical), excision of hydrocele, frenulectomy, excision of congenital sacrodermal sinus, skin lesions, muscle biopsy, anal dilatation, perianal warts, EUA, IGTN, endoscopy (gastric, rectal, colonic), excision of external angular dermoid, excision of preauricular skin tags, excision of preauricular sinus.

Urology
Cystoscopy, Sting, vulval warts, labial adhesions, circumcision, glansplasty, meatotomy, urethral dilatation, change of urinary catheter, orchidopexy, fixation of testis, some hypospadias repairs or revisions, prepucial adhesions, correction of penoscrotal web.

ENT
Myringotomy/grommets, nasal manipulation, EUA, nasal or aural foreign body removal, antral lavage, nasal cautery, evoked response audiometry, adenoidectomy*, adenotonsillectomy*.

Dental
Extractions, restorations, periodontal treatment, biopsies and minor oral surgery (e.g. mucous retention cysts), fissure sealants.

Oncology
Bone marrow sampling, lumbar puncture, intrathecal injection, node biopsy, radiotherapy, needle aspiration cytology.

Ophthalmology
EUA, measurement of IOP, probing of tear ducts, chalazion, strabismus surgery, simple skin and eyelid lesions.

Investigations
CT scans, tomography, MRI scans, blood tests, metabolic/endocrine tests, venesection.

Interventional cardiology/radiology
Balloon dilatation of strictures, transvenous occlusion of patent ductus arteriosus.

Orthopaedics
Plaster cast application and changes, arthrogram, trigger thumb, removal of sutures, injection of bone cysts, removal of metal work, excision of ganglion, removal of limb lengthening devices, minor toe surgery, biopsy, arthroscopy, intra-articular injection and minor hand surgery.

Plastic surgery
Correction of prominent ears, removal of superficial lesions, revision of scars, removal of sutures, dressing changes.

*These procedures are only carried out in some countries on a day case basis.

Table 3.2 Exclusion criteria for paediatric day case surgery

Medical exclusions	ASA Class 3*, 4, or 5
	Diabetes mellitus
	Inborn errors of metabolism
	Untreated or complex congenital heart disease
	Active viral or bacterial infection (especially upper respiratory infection)
Age exclusions	Ex-premature baby** up to 60 weeks post-conceptual age (PCA)
Anaesthetic exclusions	Inexperienced anaesthetist
	Operations of more than 1 hour's duration
	Difficult airway
	Malignant hyperpyrexia in family history
	Sibling of victims of Sudden Infant Death syndrome
	Haemoglobinopathies
Surgical exclusions	Inexperienced surgeon
	Prolonged painful procedures
	Opening of body cavity
	High risk of postoperative haemorrhage
	Adenotonsillectomy***
Social exclusions	The single parent with several children
	Poor home circumstances
	No transport
	Long distance from hospital (Greater than 1 hour travel time)

*Some ASA Class 3 patients with stable, well controlled systemic disease e.g. asthma, epilepsy, may be suitable; the healthy term neonate may be suitable.
**These babies should be categorized as ASA Class 4. Other complications of prematurity may preclude day case surgery in ex-premature babies beyond this PCA e.g. chronic lung disease (bronchopulmonary dysplasia). The healthy term neonate (0–1 month) should be considered as ASA Class 3. The healthy infant (1 month–1 yr) should be considered as ASA Class 2.
*** This operation is not recommended for day care in the UK.

Table 3.3 Advantages of paediatric day case surgery

Psychosocial	Medical	Operational
Minimal separation from parents and familiar surroundings	Reduced hospital acquired infection	Large numbers of patients can be treated
Minimal disruption to daily routine for child, parents, and other family members	Reduced respiratory complications	Reduction in waiting lists
	Reduced stress	Cost-effective
Early return to school		Concentration of
Patient preference		well trained paediatric personnel in single facility

Medical

Adult patients have a greater incidence of acquired health problems than children. Much paediatric surgery is carried out for congenital disorders in otherwise fit and healthy patients.

The American Society of Anesthesiology (ASA) classification of physical status (Table 3.4) is of value in patient selection. Most children selected for day case surgery are normal and healthy (ASA Class 1). Mild systemic disease (ASA Class 2) and well controlled, more severe disease (ASA Class 3) should not preclude day case surgery and many of these children will benefit particularly from a shortened hospital stay.

The child with mental handicap of even a severe type may be best treated in the familiar surroundings of the home. Children with well controlled epilepsy can be treated as day cases. Asthma is the most frequent disease in the paediatric population (7 per cent) and the incidence is increasing. Stress is known to trigger severe attacks and may be kept to a minimum by day care and reduced parental separation. Children with malignancy requiring investigation under anaesthesia can often be treated as day cases even in the presence of advanced disease.

Metabolic disorders contra-indicate day case surgery, because of the danger of symptomatic hypoglycaemia associated with perioperative fasting. The incidence of childhood diabetes is increasing. These children are unsuitable for day care surgery (unlike many adults) as their diabetes is always insulin dependent and frequently brittle in control.

Table 3.4 American Society of Anesthesiology classification of physical status

---

ASA Class 1
> A patient with no organic, physiological, or biochemical disturbance. The pathological process for which operation is to be performed is localized and does not entail a systemic disturbance.

ASA Class 2
> Mild to moderate systemic disturbance caused by either the condition to be treated surgically or by other pathophysiological processes.

ASA Class 3
> Severe disturbance or disease from whatever cause, even though it may not be possible to define the degree of disability with finality.

ASA Class 4
> Severe systemic disorders that are already life threatening, not always correctable by operation.

ASA Class 5
> The moribund patient who has little chance of survival but is submitted to operation in desperation.

Congenital heart disease, if untreated, is a contra-indication to most day care procedures. Children with corrected straightforward lesions such as atrial or ventricular septal defects, coarctation of the aorta, and patent ductus arteriosus may be managed on a day basis though appropriate prophylactic antibiotics may be required to prevent subacute bacterial endocarditis.

A previously undiagnosed heart murmur, even if the child is asymptomatic, must be fully investigated prior to accepting the child for day care. A paediatric cardiological opinion, echocardiography, ECG, and further investigation may be necessary.

Respiratory tract problems

The child with a runny nose may well be in the initial stages of a viral illness. Though there is no clear evidence that upper respiratory infection can lead to more severe problems, illnesses such as meningitis can present with prodromal symptoms not unlike the common cold (Berry 1990). Upper respiratory infections increase the likelihood of serious anaesthetic complications such as laryngeal spasm. This is particularly a feature after pertussis or measles as respiratory tract irritability may persist for up to six weeks (Keneally 1985).

)

Features such as purulent crusting around the nares, pyrexia, productive cough, chest signs, and lethargy should be taken into account (Levy *et al*. 1992). Thus, all children with colds or active infections should have elective surgery delayed for approximately two weeks. If lower respiratory tract signs are present, a delay of four weeks is more appropriate. The large number of children with chronic nasal discharge due to infected adenoids or allergic rhinitis may always be symptomatic and there is no benefit in delay.

Age

The ASA classification does not take age into account. However, it is reasonable to add one to the ASA class for children under 1 year (i.e. the fit infant of 9 months would be considered ASA 2) and for the healthy neonate, two should be added to the class i.e. ASA 3. In the healthy neonate, cases such as examination of the eyes for retinoblastoma, a unilateral hernia, or circumcision may be appropriate for day care provided suitably skilled paediatric anaesthetists and surgeons are involved.

The premature infant cannot be safely considered for day surgery until 60 weeks post conception. Prior to this he may be subject to life threatening apnoea following general anaesthesia and ASA class may be considered as 4 (Steward 1982). Even after 60 weeks post-conception, complications of prematurity such as chronic lung disease (bronchopulmonary dysplasia) may preclude day care. Growth retarded babies are particularly at risk from hypothermia and hypoglycaemia.

Anaesthesia

The major anaesthetic consideration for day case surgery is the brevity of the procedure. Prolonged anaesthesia usually requires prolonged recovery. Procedures taking over an hour are not generally appropriate for day care.

Procedures requiring endotracheal intubation (particularly in children under six years of age) are generally unsuitable for day care. The airway is narrow and trauma leading to even mild oedema can cause stridor. It may occur four to six hours post-extubation by which time the child may have been discharged from the hospital (Koka *et al*. 1977).

In older children the incidence of such problems is very low, provided the correct diameter of endotracheal tube is used and intubation technique is meticulous. Modern endotracheal tube materials are inherently less likely to provoke mucosal oedema. The use of the Brain laryngeal mask airway has greatly increased the safety of day case surgery around the head and neck area (Haynes and Morton 1993).

Any child with a suspected difficult airway should not be operated on as a day case, e.g. Pierre Robin, Treacher Collins, and Goldenhar syndromes. The mucopolysaccharidoses and other rare congenital disorders (Ward 1987) can cause airway problems.

Any child with a family history of malignant hyperpyrexia syndrome is not suitable for day surgery. Young children whose sibling has died from Sudden Infant Death syndrome should not be scheduled as a day case. There is no evidence to implicate anaesthesia in the syndrome, but admission for parental peace of mind is appropriate.

Any child of parents from an area of the world subject to haemoglobinopathies must be screened prior to admission. A full screen for sickle cell disease requires haemoglobin electrophoresis which takes up to 24 hours (British Society of Haematology 1988).

Surgical considerations

Much of the surgery carried out on day patients may be considered as simple, but the fact that a child is to be cared for at home requires the procedure to be done rapidly and skilfully. The trainee with little experience should not perform the operation.

The use of long acting local anaesthetics for postoperative analgesia has revolutionized the care of day patients. However, procedures requiring prolonged analgesia are not recommended for day care e.g. many orthopaedic operations. Opening a body cavity should not be done as a day care procedure. Even repair of a large umbilical hernia may lead to severe discomfort and vomiting due to air under the diaphragm. Overnight admission is advisable.

Adenotonsillectomy is frequently carried out on a day care basis in the USA. However, the current consensus of opinion in the UK is for overnight admission because of the possibility of bleeding. The maximum risk of primary haemorrhage is in the first 12 hours with an incidence of 0.47 per cent for adenoidectomy and 0.44 per cent for tonsillectomy (Capper and Randall 1984).

Preoperative preparation

Psychological

The psychological preparation of the patient and his parents should be started at the initial out-patient visit by clear information in booklet form and by discussion with nursing and medical staff. It is important for the hospital to make referring general practitioners aware of the nature and full benefits of the services provided.

Parents should be well informed about the surgical procedure, the preparations to be made, the postoperative course, and their involvement in the care of the child. A visiting community nurse can help allay parental anxieties regarding the postoperative care. The child should be given an explanation appropriate to his ability to understand. The possibility of minimizing postoperative discomfort by the use of anaesthetic creams and local anaesthetics should be mentioned.

A pre-admission programme using play simulation, photographs, books, and videos is very useful (Thornes 1991). This may be reinforced on the day of admission. The physical surroundings should be designed and decorated with children in mind. The child and parent should be encouraged to participate in the trip to the induction room. Separation from parents should be avoided. Parental presence at induction of anaesthesia is particularly beneficial to pre-school children. However, very anxious parents may be advised not to accompany their children during induction as they may transmit their anxiety to the child (Bevan *et al.* 1990).

The child should be allowed a favourite toy with him for comfort during his stay. The need for possible overnight stay must be made clear to parents before admission (Thornes 1991).

An explanatory booklet containing all the information relevant to the unit and its practices should be given to parents before admission.

Preoperative fasting

Debate continues around the length of the safe fasting period prior to general anaesthesia (Miller 1990). Prolonged fasting can lead to hypoglycaemia particularly in the child under four years of age and 15 kg body weight. It may present with overt symptoms such as impaired conscious level (commonly drowsiness) or frank convulsions. More dangerously hypoglycaemia undetected during general anaesthesia may lead to permanent neurological impairment. Most day case procedures are relatively brief and do not merit the institution of an intravenous infusion.

As important as avoiding hypoglycaemia is minimizing the risk of re-gurgitation of gastric contents and pulmonary aspiration. A compromise has to be reached.

A recent study (Farrow-Gillespie *et al.* 1988) has advocated relatively large volumes of fluid up to four hours preoperatively and claims that fluids given two hours preoperatively reduce the volume of gastric contents at the time of induction compared with fluids given four hours preoperatively. Splinter *et al.* (1989) have shown that fluids can be given safely up to two hours before anaesthesia.

The shortest possible safe period of fasting is required. Unfortunately not all age groups are alike. The **breast-fed infant** should be given a feed **four hours** before anaesthesia and nothing thereafter. The **bottle-fed infant** can be allowed **clear fluid three hours** before but milk or solid food only up to **six hours** before anaesthesia. **Older children** can be allowed a clear drink three hours before but solid food or milk no less than six hours before anaesthesia (Steward 1990).

Failure to observe the instructions regarding fasting will lead to the post-ponement or cancellation of surgery; the parents and child must understand this. As there is no nursing supervision, instructions to parents must be unequivocal (Table 3.5).

However, it must also be made clear that prolonged starvation can be harmful. Children presenting for an afternoon list should not be starved from the previous evening. In a recent clinical audit of 207 paediatric day cases, there were two cases of symptomatic hypoglycaemia due to prolonged fasting (Stuart and Morton 1991). Hypoglycaemia is therefore very infrequent with fewer than 1 per cent of cases requiring intravenous glucose. Unfortunately, some mothers who have fasted with their child have also had to be treated for hypoglycaemia.

Admission procedure

On admission, the child should be examined to exclude any recent additional physical signs and a history regarding fasting must be taken. The child must be weighed and his temperature taken. Routine haemoglobin estimation and chest X-ray are not necessary.

The child should not be obliged to change into hospital clothing and there is no need to confine him to bed. The environment should be as friendly and familiar as possible with the accent on play and activities such as television, videos, books, and toys.

Premedication

Most day case patients are not given sedative premedication, particularly if parents are accompanying them during the induction of anaesthesia. However, some children who attend regularly (for example for repeat examinations for retinoblastoma, glaucoma, or urethral dilatation) may benefit from a mild sedative. This should not be withheld simply because of the nature of day case procedures. Traditional oral sedatives are long acting and may delay recovery, and narcotic premedication increases the incidence of nausea and vomiting to levels which increase the overnight admission rate. Oral midazolam, 0.5–0.7 mg/kg, produces useful sedation within 30 minutes without prolonging recovery. It has a bitter taste, however, which must be disguised by mixing with a sweet drink.

Occasionally, a very difficult or uncooperative child may require, with parental consent, a last minute premedication with rapidly acting agents. Intramuscular ketamine, 2 mg/kg acts in 2–3 minutes and allows separation of the child from his parent and application of a face mask for inhalational induction to continue. Recovery is not prolonged by this relatively small dose of ketamine.

Table 3.5 An example of preoperative parental instructions for a child attending for day surgery at 12.30

ROYAL HOSPITAL FOR SICK CHILDREN DAY SURGERY UNIT
PARENT'S GUIDE (AFTERNOON SURGERY)

Dear ....

Please bring .... to the Day Surgery Unit at

11.00 am on ....

If .... has a cold or other illness please telephone
041-339-8888, extension 4108, between 8.30 am and 5.00 pm.

.... should have a bath, shower or wash before
coming to the Day Surgery Unit.

*************************** **IMPORTANT** ****************************

.... must have **NO** food, milk or milky drinks after 6.30 am.
A drink of juice or water should be encouraged up to 9.30 am. After that time
he/she should have **NO** food or drink.

If your child is breast fed, the last feed should be at 8.30 am.

You should understand that for safety reasons the surgery will
be postponed or cancelled if you do not follow these instructions.

You should expect to spend at least 5 hours in the hospital.

Checklist:		
	No food after	6.30am
	No milky drinks after	6.30am
	No bottle milk after	6.30am
	No breast milk after	8.30am
	Encourage juice/water up to	9.30am

Alternative techniques for this situation in pre-school children are intra-nasal midazolam, 0.2 mg/kg, or rectal methohexitone, 25 mg/kg (10% solution). Both will produce adequate sedation within 10 minutes in the majority of children without delaying recovery significantly.

Local anaesthetic cream (EMLA Astra) should be applied under an occlusive dressing as a routine on admission, to allow at least one hour for the cream to take its full effect. The site(s) of application are selected by the anaesthetist or a trained nurse. The ester local anaesthetic amethocaine, in a gel or transdermal patch formulation, offers an alternative (Coley 1989; Freeman *et al.* 1993).

Antibiotic cover for congenital cardiac defects and steroid cover for dependent patients is administered intravenously following induction.

Patients taking routine medication (such as inhalers for asthma) should be allowed these at the normal times and should bring any such drugs with them to the hospital on the day of surgery.

References

Berry, F. A. (1990). The child with the runny nose. In *Anesthetic management of the difficult and routine patient*, (2nd edn), (ed. F. A. Berry), pp. 267–83. Churchill Livingstone, New York.

Bevan, J. C., Johnston, C., Haig, M. J., Tousignant, G., Lucy, S., Kirnon, V., *et al.* (1990). Pre-operative parental anxiety predicts behavioural and emotional responses to induction of anaesthesia in children. *Canadian Journal of Anaesthesia*, **37**, 177–82.

British Society of Haematology (1988). Guidelines for haemoglobinopathy screening. *Clinics in Laboratory Haematology*, **10**, 87–94.

Capper, J. W. R. and Randall, C. (1984). Post-operative haemorrhage in tonsillectomy and adenoidectomy in children. *Journal of Laryngology and Otology*, **98**, 363–5.

Coley, S. (1989). Anaesthesia of the skin. *British Journal of Anaesthesia*, **62**, 4–5.

Farrow-Gillespie, A., Christensen, S., and Lerman, J. (1988). Effect of the fasting interval on gastric pH and volume in children. *Anesthesia and Analgesia*, **67**, S59.

Freeman, J. A., Doyle, E., Ng, T. I., and Morton, N. S. (1993). Topical anaesthesia of the skin: a review. *Paediatric Anaesthesia*, **3**, 129–38.

Haynes, S. R. and Morton, N. S. (1993). The laryngeal mask airway: a review of its use in paediatric anaesthesia. *Paediatric Anaesthesia*, **3**, 65–73.

Keneally, J. P. (1985). Day stay surgery in paediatrics. *Clinics in Anesthesiology*, **3**, 679–96.

Koka, B. V., Jeon, I. S., and Andre, J. M. (1977). Post-intubation croup in children. *Anesthesia and Analgesia*, **56**, 501.

Levy, L., Pandit, U. A., Randel, G. I., Lewis, I. H., and Tait, A. R. (1992). Upper respiratory tract infections and general anaesthesia in children. Peri-operative complications and oxygen saturation. *Anaesthesia*, **47**, 678–82.

Miller, D. C. (1990). Why are children starved? *British Journal of Anaesthesia*, **64**, 409–10.

Splinter, W. M., Stewart, J. A., and Muir, J. G. (1989). The effect of pre-operative apple juice on gastric contents, thirst and hunger in children. *Canadian Journal of Anaesthesia*, **36**, 55–8.

Steward, D. J. (1982). Preterm infants are more prone to complications following minor surgery than are term infants. *Anesthesiology*, **56**, 304–6.

Steward, D. J. (1990). Getting ready for day care. In *Outpatient anesthesia*, (ed. P. F. White), pp. 177–8. Churchill Livingstone, New York.

Stuart, J. C. and Morton, N. S. (1991). A clinical audit of day case surgery for children. *Journal of One Day Surgery*, **1**, 15–8.

Thomas, D. K. M. (1974). Hypoglycaemia in children before operation, its incidence and prevention. *British Journal of Anaesthesia*, **46**, 66–8.

Thornes, R. (1991). *Just for the day*. NAWCH Ltd, London.

Ward, C. F. (1987). Pediatric head and neck syndromes. In *Anesthesia and uncommon pediatric diseases*, (ed. J. Katz and D. J. Steward). W. B. Saunders, Philadelphia.

4 Anaesthetic management

INDUCTION OF ANAESTHESIA

N. S. Morton

Intravenous induction of anaesthesia has been revolutionized by the routine use of topical anaesthesia of the skin (Coley 1989). Some anaesthetists favour winged needle devices or the use of very small needles (25 or 27 gauge) for the initial injection. Most now favour the immediate placement of an indwelling intravenous cannula (22 or 24 gauge) with a capped injection port. The dorsum of the hand is the most often used site where painless cannulation can be achieved in up to 96 per cent of children with EMLA cream preparation.

The choice of agent for intravenous induction of paediatric day cases rests between propofol and thiopentone in modern practice. Propofol has been shown to produce rapid, smooth induction with a low incidence of serious adverse effects (Morton *et al.* 1992). Recovery is quicker and of better quality in children as in adults after propofol compared with thiopentone (Puttick and Rosen 1988; Mirakhur 1988; Runcie *et al.* 1993).

Pain on injection can occur with both agents (Morton *et al.* 1988). The addition of lignocaine to propofol immediately prior to injection is well recognized in adults to abolish injection pain and is effective when the veins on the dorsum of the hand are used in children (Morton 1990). The minimum effective dose of lignocaine for this purpose in children is 0.2 mg/kg when added to 3 mg/kg of propofol (Cameron *et al.* 1992).

The dose requirement for propofol is higher in unpremedicated children than in adults because the volume of the central compartment is 50 per cent larger, and the clearance is 25 per cent higher in children. Thus 3–4 mg/kg is the usual induction dose (Morton *et al.* 1992).

Thiopentone 5–6 mg/kg is a satisfactory induction agent in unpremedicated children (Cote *et al.* 1981). Dose related cardiovascular effects are seen, with both agents causing a fall in blood pressure, while thiopentone causes a rise in heart rate and propofol a fall in heart rate (Morton *et al.* 1988; Short and Aun 1991). Halothane potentiates the fall in heart rate seen with propofol and operations involving a parasympathetic stimulus (e.g. orchidopexy, herniotomy) warrant extra vigilance as significant bradycardia and hypotension may occur.

Involuntary movements may be seen with propofol induction in children, which may be alarming to accompanying parents. They are invariably associated with the use of an inadequate induction dose and too early stimulation of the child (Borgeat *et al.* 1991; Borgeat and Wilder-Smith 1991). A supplemental dose of 0.5 mg/kg propofol and gentle application of the face mask and jaw support can avoid this problem. In our unit, propofol has superseded thiopentone for induction of paediatric day cases (Stuart and Morton 1991).

Inhalational induction may be preferred where difficulty with venous access is anticipated, or when a child specifically requests it. In older co-operative children, the single vital capacity breath method can be used (Lamberty and Wilson 1987; Loper *et al.* 1987; Drummond 1988; MacKenzie 1990).

For inhalational induction, halothane remains the agent of choice, producing the most rapid induction (Simmons *et al.* 1989) with the least respiratory side effects (Sampaio *et al.* 1989) and remarkable cardiovascular stability (Morton *et al.* 1988). Desflurane, though theoretically attractive, in practice produces excessive adverse respiratory effects (Zwass *et al.* 1992). Sevoflurane produces a rapid, smooth inhalational induction rivalling halothane in its lack of irritant airways effects and may find a place in paediatric day case anaesthesia in the future (Lerman 1992).

Other occasionally used techniques of induction include rectal administration of benzodiazepines or barbiturates, or intramuscular administration of ketamine, or intranasal midazolam (see Chapter 3).

The logistics of the induction should be flexible for each patient and accompanying parent. Small children prefer to be in their parent's arms or on their lap, while older children may prefer to sit or lie on a trolley with their parent close by. This degree of flexibility is possible in a fully equipped induction room.

MAINTENANCE OF ANAESTHESIA

N. S. Morton

For most day case surgical procedures in children, spontaneous respiration of nitrous oxide, oxygen, and a volatile anaesthetic agent via a clear, soft rimmed face mask or via a laryngeal mask airway (LMA) is satisfactory (Haynes and Morton 1993). The LMA has the advantage of providing a secure airway while freeing the anaesthetist to carry out a local anaesthetic nerve block for example. The size 2 LMA is used in up to 55 per cent of paediatric day cases in our unit (Stuart and Morton 1991). LMA insertion is easier after propofol induction (McGinn *et al.* 1993). The insertion technique described by McNicol (1991) is very useful (Fig. 4.1). The LMA is inserted with the aperture facing cephalad initially until the tip of the mask is beyond the base of the tongue. Then as the LMA is advanced, it is rotated 180° anti-clockwise until the aperture is aligned with the laryngeal inlet.

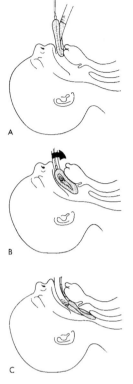

Fig. 4.1 Rotational technique of insertion of LMA in children (McNicol 1991)

A

B

C

Recently maintenance of anaesthesia with propofol by infusion has been described and produces similar cardiovascular and respiratory effects to halothane maintenance with similar recovery times (Doyle *et al.* 1993).

Endotracheal intubation is seldom required other than in an emergency or where determined by the operative procedure. Suxamethonium should be avoided where possible in ambulant children, as it may cause muscle pains (Bush and Roth 1961; Lyle 1982; Stuart and Morton 1991), although these are less common in younger children. Intubation can be facilitated by deep halothane anaesthesia, by alfentanil or by use of a small dose of non-depolarizing muscle relaxant. Sore throat and post-extubation subglottic oedema with stridor can be minimized by careful technique, and by choosing the correct size of endotracheal tube (i.e. one where a demonstrable leak can be heard when an airway pressure of 20 cm H_2O is applied). Should stridor occur, humidity, dexamethasone (0.6 mg/kg IV), and nebulized adrenaline (0.5 ml/kg/dose of 1:1000, max. 5 mls) are recognized treatments. If stridor persists for more than four hours, or in any cases of doubt, the child should be admitted for observation to a High Dependency Unit or Intensive Care Unit.

Intra-operative monitoring

The most important monitor is that provided by the continuous presence of a senior anaesthetist, using his/her clinical skills to assess the adequacy of the child's respiration, perfusion, analgesia, and anaesthesia. A precordial stethoscope is a useful non-invasive monitor but electronic monitoring to the same standard as in-patient operating theatres is essential (i.e. electrocardiograph, pulse oximeter, automated non-invasive blood pressure recorder, temperature probe). Capnography is useful although interpretation can be difficult in paediatrics (Stokes and Clutton-Brock 1990). A defibrillator and the full range of resuscitation equipment and drugs must be immediately to hand.

LOCAL ANAESTHESIA

L. R. McNicol

Rationale for local anaesthesia

Local anaesthesia is used in paediatric practice to prevent acute pain, most commonly to relieve postoperative pain. Various techniques can be used as part of a balanced anaesthetic if administered after the induction of anaesthesia (Arthur and McNicol 1986). As a result general anaesthetic requirements can be reduced as the block becomes established. Depending on the type of block used, postoperative analgesia of varying degrees and duration can be produced.

Many of the benefits attributed to the use of intraoperative local anaesthesia are in fact due to the lack of side effects when compared with alternative techniques. Either no postoperative analgesia is given or minor oral analgesic preparations such as paracetamol or major systemic analgesics such as the opioids may be used. The problems associated with these techniques are inadequate relief of pain (of varying degrees) or the well known side effects of opioid analgesia (nausea, vomiting, anorexia, and central sedation). Cohen *et al.* (1990) recently reviewed the perianaesthetic complications associated with over 20 000 paediatric anaesthetics. Nausea and vomiting occurred in over 30 per cent of these anaesthetics, being mainly associated with the use of opioid analgesics. Many children also had inadequate relief of pain. These authors were so concerned at the scale of these side effects, that they changed their anaesthetic techniques during the period of the audit, local anaesthesia being substituted for opioid analgesia as part of a balanced anaesthetic technique. Thus, the judicious and appropriate use of local anaesthesia can prevent many of these complications and children will waken rapidly following their anaesthetic with either no pain, or minimal pain and little gastrointestinal upset. Fluids and food will rapidly be accepted, ambulation will be commenced early and discharge will not be delayed.

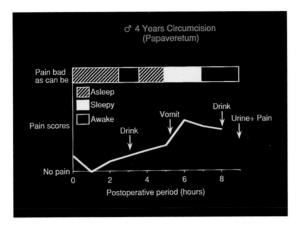

Fig. 4.2a Postoperative pain profile of a boy following circumcision. Analgesia consisted of intravenous and intramuscular papavaratum administered after the induction of anaesthesia

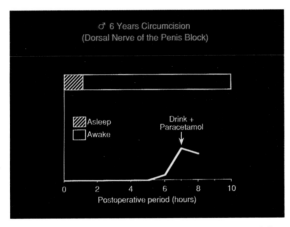

Fig. 4.2b Postoperative pain profile of a boy following circumcision. Postoperative analgesia consisted of a block of the dorsal nerve of the penis after the induction of anaesthesia

Figure 4.2 demonstrates the advantages of the use of pre-emptive local anaesthesia in individual patients on whom circumcisions were performed on an in-patient basis. Both patients (1*a* and 1*b*) had similar anaesthetics, the main difference being that patient (a) received papaveratum 1 mg per 3 kg of body weight, half given intravenously and half intramuscularly at the induction of anaesthesia and patient (b) received a block of the dorsal nerve of the penis using 0.5% bupivacaine. In the early postoperative period, both patients had their pain assessed by the same nurse using a visual linear analogue scale, 0 being 'no pain' and 10 being 'pain as bad as can be'. The postoperative pain profile of patient (a) shows many of the drawbacks of opioid analgesia, i.e. inadequate pain relief, pain relief at the expense of central sedation, and gastrointestinal dysfunction. Patient (b) was assessed as having no pain for many hours into the postoperative period; there was little central sedation; he ate and drank liberally and was up and running about the ward not long after his return from the operating theatre. This pattern can be repeated using other nerve blocks.

Sites for administration of local anaesthetic

It is possible to reversibly block transmission of painful stimuli by applying local anaesthetic agents at a variety of sites as shown in Fig. 4.3.

Stimuli originating from mucous membranes can be prevented by the use of topical local anaesthesia. Simple infiltration anaesthesia is especially useful for very superficial lesions of the skin and can be injected into the deeper layers of wounds intraoperatively. Small distal peripheral nerves, frequently the anterior cutaneous branches of the ventral rami, can be blocked to produce areas of analgesia while avoiding weakness of associated muscles. Proximal blocks of larger nerves, although possible, are best not performed on patients undergoing day care surgery, as the associated loss of motor power can be very trouble-some. Central blocks—commonly caudal extradural block—can be performed on out-patients, although most paediatric anaesthetists would rather perform a peripheral nerve block as an alternative.

Possible sites for Application of Local Anaesthetics

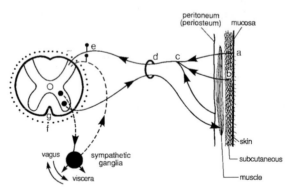

Fig. 4.3 Simplified diagram of nerve pathways showing sites for administration of local anaesthetic: a: topical analgesia; b: subcutaneous infiltration; c: distal sensory nerve block; d: proximal mixed peripheral nerve block; e: paravertebral block; f: extradural block; g: subarachnoid block. Note that e, f, and g also block the sympathetic system thus modifying visceral pain and causing peripheral vasodilation.

Choice of local anaesthetic agent

1. Bupivacaine

Although many local anaesthetic agents are available for producing analgesia, at a practical level only one is commonly used. Bupivacaine is an amide local anaesthetic and virtually all studies investigating the efficacy of various peripheral nerve blocks in paediatric practice have been carried out using this drug as the local anaesthetic agent.

The onset of action of bupivacaine is longer than other local anaesthetic agents which is acceptable in the light of its long duration of action. Surgical anaesthesia varying from three to ten hours is produced depending on the block. The addition of adrenaline does prolong the duration of action of bupivacaine when it is used for infiltration and blocks of peripheral nerves, but not as dramatically as with the shorter acting local anaesthetic agents such as lignocaine.

Bupivacaine is available in several strengths, although only the 0.5% (5 mg/ml) and the 0.25% (2.5 mg/ml) solutions are commonly used. Bupivacaine 0.5% is equivalent in potency to lignocaine 2.0% and can be used mainly for blocking individual nerves but also in appropriate dosage for small areas of local infiltration. Bupivacaine 0.25% is the concentration of choice when widespread local infiltration is used.

Dose of bupivacaine

The recommended maximum dose of bupivacaine is 2 mg/kg of body weight. Higher doses have been administered to children without clinical signs of toxicity or maximum peak drug concentration (C_{max}) reaching 2–4 μg/ml, which may cause CNS toxicity in adults. C_{max} and T_{max} (time to maximal blood level of local anaesthetic) depend on other factors apart from the total dose of bupivacaine administered, not least of which is the age of the patient.

Effect of age

Neonates and infants may be at increased risk of toxic effects of amide local anaesthetics because of lower levels of albumin and alpha-1-acid glycoprotein (AAG), both proteins being important for the binding of local anaesthetics. Their binding properties are very different, albumin having a low affinity for local anaesthetics and almost never becoming saturated. AAG has a high affinity for these drugs and a greater number of molecules can be bound per mole compared to albumin. AAG soon becomes saturated, and once this threshold is reached the free fraction of drug increases very rapidly when the total concentration in the plasma increases. Both these protein levels are very low at birth, albumin being 60–80% of adult levels and AAG 50%. Adult levels are not reached until between six and twelve months of age.

Mazoit *et al.* (1986) showed that following the caudal administration of bupivacaine, the free fraction of this drug was increased in infants at least until six months of age. These workers also showed an inverse relationship between the free fraction of bupivacaine and age parallel to the decrease in AAG concentrations and age.

Other factors which influence protein binding, apart from age, include metabolic and respiratory acidosis which increases the free fraction of bupivacaine. An anaesthetic technique associated with under ventilation of a small infant may lead to a sudden increase in the risk of toxicity of local anaesthetics. Although neonates are not generally admitted for day case surgery, they are especially at risk if suffering from jaundice as bilirubin competes with bupivacaine for albumin resulting in higher free levels of this anaesthetic agent.

Effect of site of injection

C_{max} and T_{max} also depend on the sites of injection of bupivacaine. Tucker and Mather (1979, 1986) have shown in adults that the rate of absorption of local anaesthetic agents decreases in the order intercostal, caudal, extradural, brachial plexus, and sciatico-femoral. In paediatric practice few controlled studies have been carried out comparing C_{max} and T_{max} from different sites of injection. However, with a few exceptions, blood levels in children tend to follow the same pattern as found in adults, with C_{max} of bupivacaine decreasing in the order intrapleural, intercostal, caudal, extradural, and iliohypogastric/ilioinguinal and subcutaneous infiltration. Although differences in absorption rates as a function of concentration of drug used, volume of injection, and speed of injection have been described, it is doubtful if they affect C_{max} and T_{max} significantly. The addition of adrenaline to local anaesthetic agents (usually in the proportion of 1 in 200 000) decreases C_{max} after most of the common regional blocks although it does not always prolong T_{max}. This suggests that although the mean absorption time is increased, a proportion of local anaesthetic is still rapidly absorbed before vasoconstriction is complete. In general, the beneficial effects of adrenaline are seen after blocks associated with high C_{max} and with the shorter acting local anaesthetic agents rather than longer acting anaesthetic agents such as bupivacaine.

Toxicity

Cardiovascular and CNS system toxicity have rarely been observed in children following local anaesthetic administration. Convulsions are rarely noted as their seizure threshold may be increased by the use of general anaesthetics or sedatives. Badgwell *et al.* (1990) investigated bupivacaine toxicity in young pigs, whose cardiovascular systems are very similar to those of humans, and they concluded that nitrous oxide anaesthesia plus halothane or isoflurane increases the lethality of bupivacaine by depressing the cardiac index while preventing early warning signs of toxicity i.e. convulsions.

The treatment of toxic reactions to local anaesthetics is the same as with any anaesthetic emergency. Initial treatment should be aimed at oxygenating the patient adequately with priority being given to maintaining the airway, ensuring adequate ventilation and supporting circulation. Even a short period of convulsions may have catastrophic effects if a child is allowed to become acidotic and hypercarbic. The resultant increase in free local anaesthetic and cerebral perfusion produces an increased uptake of local anaesthetic agent by the brain. Convulsions are best controlled with a benzodiazepine, but when taking place in an anaesthetic room or operating theatre, thiopentone is often available and is a potent alternative.

The concept of 'maximum allowable dose' of bupivacaine is a complicated one because of the many factors mentioned above, and any suggested upper limits have to be given assuming that the drug has been administered correctly. For instance, a small dose of bupivacaine carelessly or inadvertently injected into a blood vessel, could result in serious side effects, whereas a 'maximum allowable dose' injected slowly into an area of low vascularity, for example subcutaneously, may result in blood levels well below the assumed toxic levels.

2. Lignocaine

Although bupivacaine is by far the most commonly used local anaesthetic agent for paediatric day case surgery, different preparations of other local anaesthetics do have a role. Lignocaine is the most versatile of these agents and can be used for topical anaesthesia in the form of a 2% gel, a 5% ointment, or 10% aerosol. Solutions of 0.5%, 1%, 1.5%, and 2% are available for infiltration and nerve block. Lignocaine has a rapid onset and moderate duration of action lasting approximately two hours for various regional anaesthetic procedures. Preparations containing adrenaline last significantly longer and in addition the rate of absorption of the drug is significantly decreased as is its potential for producing systemic toxic reactions.

3. Amethocaine

The only ester type of local anaesthetic used regularly is amethocaine, which is used for topical anaesthesia of the conjunctiva and cornea. Although this agent has the potential for systemic toxic reactions when large doses are used, it is quite safe to use either a 0.5% or 1% solution in the volumes required for ophthalmic procedures. A gel formulation is being developed for anaesthesia of the skin (Freeman *et al.* 1993).

4. Prilocaine

Prilocaine is an amide local anaesthetic with a clinical profile similar to that of lignocaine. In combination with lignocaine as a eutectic mixture of local anaesthetic agents (EMLA) prilocaine has found a new life as a topical local anaesthetic agent, providing analgesia for simple but important procedures such as venepuncture. Prilocaine cannot be recommended for use in neonates and small infants because of the risks of methaemoglobinaemia which although rarely of clinical significance, can confuse the aetiology of cyanosis. As the least toxic of the local amide anaesthetic agents, prilocaine is particularly useful for intravenous regional anaesthesia (Bier's block).

Although the use of local anaesthesia in general has many advantages over conventional techniques of producing intra- and postoperative analgesia there are certain disadvantages which have to be considered. Many blocks are relatively simple and can be learned quickly but others do require a degree of expertise which may take some time to develop. Fortunately the nature of the operative procedures carried out on out-patient children is such that only simple local anaesthetic techniques need to be mastered. However, it is the practice of some paediatric anaesthetists still to perform more complicated blocks, such as caudal extradural blocks which require proper training and experience for their success. Extra time is also required for more complicated blocks and this can cause problems during busy operating sessions.

The following description of the techniques of specific nerve blocks will commence with those acting most peripherally (e.g. topical anaesthesia) and will proceed proximally, ending with caudal extradural block.

Topical anaesthesia

This is a simple method of producing good analgesia which, depending on the operative procedure, can last for two or more hours. If an oral analgesic such as paracetamol or dihydrocodeine is administered before the block wears off, it is possible to take patients through the early part of the postoperative period without having to endure severe pain.

Eutectic mixture of local anaesthetics (EMLA)

The term 'eutectic mixture' describes the phenomenon noted when two solids undergo a phase change to a liquid. Thus a 1:1 mixture of solid crystalline lignocaine and prilocaine form a eutectic which is a liquid at room temperature. EMLA cream (Astra pharmaceuticals) comprises lignocaine (25 mg/ml), prilocaine (25 mg/ml), Arlatone (an emulsifier), and Carbopol (a thickener).

When applied to the skin and covered by an occlusive dressing (Fig. 4.4) superficial analgesia can be produced which can be useful for a number of minor procedures. By far the most important of these is relief of the pain associated with venepuncture. Fear of needles and injections is a common source of children's unhappiness when admitted to hospital, and this can be allayed in most children when it is explained to them that the 'magic cream' will mean that they should feel no pain during the insertion of a needle. Figure 4.5 shows a typical reaction following the insertion of a cannula prior to induction of

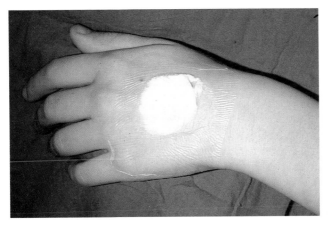

Fig. 4.4 Eutectic mixture of local anaesthetics (EMLA) cream applied to dorsum of hand prior to venepuncture

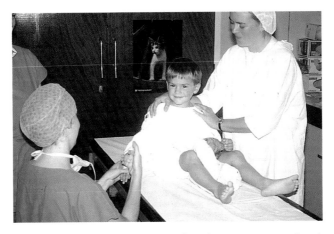

Fig. 4.5 Typical child following insertion of an intravenous cannula when EMLA cream is applied at the site of injection 1.5 hours beforehand

anaesthesia. The demeanour of the child shown in the illustration changed little during insertion of a cannula.

It has to be stressed that EMLA cream should be administered a minimum of 1 hour, and preferably longer, before venepuncture to be wholly effective. One-quarter to one-fifth of a 5 g tube is a suitable dose. Following removal of EMLA cream it is not uncommon to find an area of pallor with associated vasoconstriction of veins in this area and this can sometimes make insertion of a cannula difficult as there is often no 'flash-back' of blood when the cannula enters the vein. However, if the EMLA cream is removed about 10 minutes before the venepuncture, the skin and blood vessels revert to normal. Many children do not react to the needle passing through the skin during venepuncture but are aware of a sensation as the needle point enters the vein. It is worth explaining this to older children who may be taken by surprise and whose confidence may suffer as a result.

EMLA cream can also be used prior to the injection of local anaesthetic in older children undergoing minor superficial surgical procedures without recourse to general anaesthesia. This is a useful addition to the anaesthetist's armamentarium for day case surgery as many surgical procedures lend themselves to this technique in appropriate children. Even younger children, from seven years old, will allow minor surgery to be performed if a gentle confident

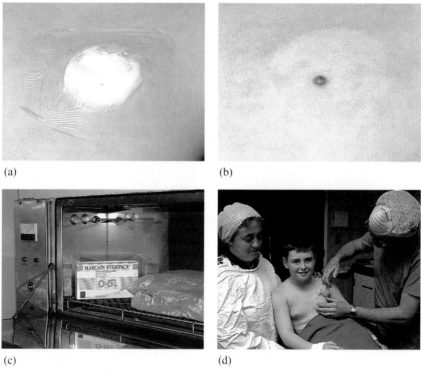

(a)   (b)

(c)   (d)

Fig. 4.6 The use of EMLA cream as part of a local anaesthetic technique without recourse to general anaesthesia. (a) One-quarter of a tube of EMLA cream is applied over the lesion 1.5–2 hours preoperatively. (b) the EMLA cream has been removed and an area of vasoconstriction and pallor can be seen around the lesion. (c) Bupivacaine 0.5% with adrenaline is removed from the warm cabinet. (d) Bupivacaine is slowly injected using a fine needle.

technique as described in Fig. 4.6 is used. The removal of naevi, warts, and *molluscum contagiosum* are typical examples of the kind of surgery that can be carried out using this technique. Although patients generally do not complain when the needle penetrates the skin they often complain of slight discomfort when the local anaesthetic is injected and this can be minimized by warming the bupivacaine to body temperature prior to injecting it, using a fine needle e.g. 25 gauge, and by injecting the bupivacaine very slowly.

The division of foreskin adhesions is a minor procedure with enough discomfort to warrant recourse to general anaesthesia. However, if EMLA cream is applied to the foreskin under an occlusive dressing and allowed to penetrate down to the region of the glans penis these adhesions can be divided while the child is still conscious if a gentle confident approach is used by the surgeon.

Mucosal analgesia

Although squint surgery is not carried out wholly on out-patients in the UK, there is an increasing tendency for this to happen and good quality postoperative analgesia without recourse to potent analgesics is therefore an important part of the anaesthetic. This can be achieved by instilling 1% amethocaine eyedrops into the conjunctival sac at the conclusion of surgery but before the patient recovers from anaesthesia (Fig. 4.7). Good quality postoperative analgesia lasting two to three hours is produced during which time it is possible to administer a simple oral analgesic such as paracetamol or dihydrocodeine (Watson 1991).

When squint surgery is carried out using conventional general anaesthetic techniques there is a high incidence of postoperative nausea and vomiting.

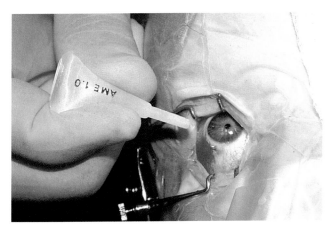

Fig. 4.7 Topical anaesthesia following squint surgery. Amethocaine eyedrops 1% are instilled into the conjunctival sac at the completion of surgery

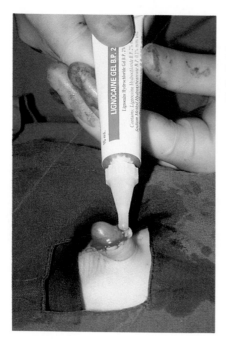

Fig. 4.8 Application of lignocaine gel to the penis after circumcision. Parents can be taught to repeat this procedure at home during the first postoperative day

50–80 per cent of children may be affected by this, possibly as a result of an oculo-emetic reflex, and it is the author's experience over many years that the use of topical amethocaine can dramatically reduce these unfortunate postoperative sequelae.

Lignocaine preparations can be used topically to produce postoperative pain relief for some common out-patient operative procedures. The pain following an anal stretch carried out in children suffering from anal fissures can be dramatically relieved by the application of 2% lignocaine jelly or 5% lignocaine ointment at the conclusion of surgery. More importantly, the pain associated with circumcision can be dramatically modified by the use of topically applied lignocaine (Fig. 4.8). Tree-Trakarn and Pirayavaraporn (1985) used various preparations of lignocaine applied topically to prevent postoperative pain following circumcision—10% lignocaine spray applied as a thin film or 0.5–1 ml of either 5% lignocaine ointment or 2% lignocaine gel. These techniques provided postoperative analgesia equal to morphine or to a block of the dorsal nerve of the penis. The complications of the latter two techniques, namely central sedation, nausea, vomiting, or failure are thus avoided. It is important to remember that the lignocaine preparation should be applied at the conclusion of surgery before the patient recovers consciousness. It is less effective to use this technique if the patient is awake and complaining of pain.

Instillation of local anaesthetic

This is a simple technique which is non-invasive, safe, and can achieve a moderate degree of postoperative analgesia. Casey *et al.* (1990) compared children who had 0.25% bupivacaine in a dose of 0.25 ml/kg instilled into their wounds during repair of inguinal hernia under general anaesthesia with a group of children who had iliohypogastric/ilioinguinal nerve blocks and found little difference between the two groups. This technique does not provide any degree of intraoperative analgesia and it is the author's experience that instillation of local anaesthetics does not last as long as a peripheral nerve block.

Infiltration of local anaesthetic agents

Infiltration anaesthesia is commonly carried out in children for simple surgical procedures, such as the suturing of lacerations. However, if performed by surgeons intraoperatively before the wound is closed or, in some cases after the wound is closed, a degree of postoperative analgesia can be achieved which again is effective, non-invasive, and safe. It is important to be aware that this technique can involve large volumes of local anaesthetic compared to blocks of peripheral nerves where a small volume of local anaesthetic can be accurately placed close to a nerve. Due consideration must be given to the maturity and weight of the patients to prevent inadvertent overdose of local anaesthetic. Virtually any surgical procedure carried out on paediatric out-patients is suitable for this technique as most are of a minor nature and commonly superficial. It is especially useful for excision of 'lumps and bumps', for example dermoid cysts, sebaceous cysts, and accessory auricles. If bupivacaine 0.5% with adrenaline is injected following release of tongue-ties in a dose of about 0.5−1 ml, complete and long lasting postoperative analgesia can be achieved (Fig. 4.9). If superficial skin lesions such as naevi are infiltrated with bupivacaine 0.5% with adrenaline following induction of anaesthesia good intraoperative haemostasis can be achieved as well as good postoperative analgesia (Fig. 4.10).

Inguinal hernia repair is a common procedure carried out on children on an out-patient basis and simple wound infiltration is a well recognized method of producing postoperative analgesia. Fell *et al.* (1988) produced analgesia using this technique comparable with that of a caudal extradural block and Reid *et al.* (1987) produced analgesia equal to that of a block of the iliohypogastric and ilioinguinal nerves. Mobley *et al.* (1991) studied a group of children in whom the wound edges were infiltrated with 1.25 mg/kg of bupivacaine without adrenaline. Children under 16 kg received the 0.25% solution and older children the 0.5% solution. These authors found that the mean C_{max} was 0.35 μg/ml at T_{max} of 14.6 minutes after infiltration, i.e. much lower than the proposed

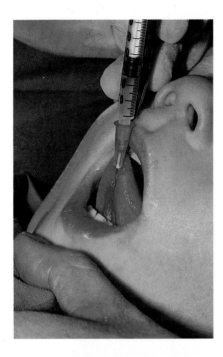

Fig. 4.9 Infiltration local anaesthesia for release of tongue-tie. 0.5−1 ml of 0.5% bupivacaine are injected into the wound before the patient recovers from anaesthesia

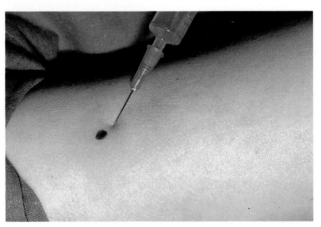

Fig. 4.10 Infiltration anaesthesia for removal of skin lesion. 2 ml of 0.5% bupivacaine with adrenaline are injected subcutaneously after the induction of anaesthesia around a pigmented lesion of skin. As well as providing good postoperative analgesia this also causes vasoconstriction and prevents intraoperative bleeding

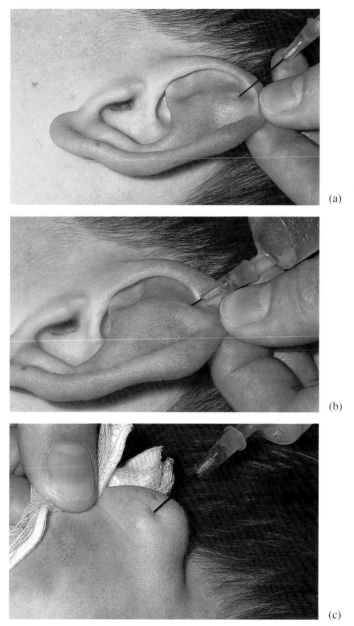

(a)

(b)

(c)

Fig. 4.11 Subcutaneous infiltration for correction of prominent ears. (a) A fine needle is inserted subcutaneously on the outer surface of the ear. (b) 0.25% bupivacaine and hyaluronidase are injected and spread rapidly throughout the subcutaneous structures of the ear. (c) This is repeated on the inner surface of the ear

concentration of 2—4 μg/ml which may be associated with the onset of CNS toxicity in adults.

The operation of otoplasty (correction of prominent ears) is one of the most commonly performed plastic surgical procedures in paediatric practice and is frequently carried out on an out-patient basis. This procedure is associated with severe pain and there is an increased incidence of nausea and vomiting especially if systemic analgesics are used on their own. Good analgesia can be produced postoperatively using a small volume of local anaesthetic if the great auricular nerve is blocked. However, an alternative is to use bupivacaine with adrenaline for subcutaneous infiltration of the ears to a total dose of 2 mg/kg. Not only will this produce postoperative analgesia of moderate duration but the associated vasoconstriction produces haemostasis and good operating conditions. If hyaluronidase is added to the local anaesthetic solution in a ratio of about 1500 international units to 20 ml of local anaesthetic the solution rapidly spreads from one single point of injection ensuring a more efficient block without multiple puncture sites on the ear (Fig. 4.11).

Peripheral nerve blocks

For surgery in the inguinal region

Figure 4.12 shows the cutaneous distribution of the nerves originating from the nerve root LI—the iliohypogastric nerve and the ilioinguinal nerve. The iliohypogastric nerve is by far the more important of these and may be thought of as the 'thirteenth intercostal nerve' and indeed in about 50 per cent of patients it is accompanied by the twelfth intercostal nerve—the subcostal nerve. Although the iliohypogastric nerve supplies branches to muscle and parietal peritoneum, at the level of the anterior superior iliac spine only the anterior cutaneous branch can be blocked thus preventing pain arising from skin and subcutaneous tissues. However, this is sufficient to provide good postoperative analgesia following the repair of inguinal hernia, since only the very superficial layers of the abdominal wall are operated on during this procedure especially in young children.

In older children (above two years of age) many surgeons open up the inguinal canal to locate the sac of the inguinal hernia which is supplied by the ilioinguinal nerve. This nerve courses through the loin between the external and internal oblique muscles. It lies beneath the external oblique aponeurosis just medial to the anterior superior iliac spine. This nerve also supplies the upper innermost part of the thigh and the anterior part of the scrotum in boys and of the *mons pubis* in girls. Thus it can be seen that for good postoperative analgesia both the iliohypogastric and ilioinguinal nerves have to blocked.

In the proximal part of its course the iliohypogastric nerve runs between the transversus muscle and the internal oblique muscle, it pierces the latter again just

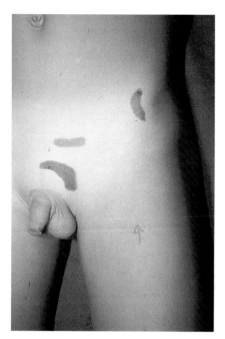

Fig. 4.12 Innervation of nerves from spinal route LI. The pale untanned 'underpant' area corresponds to the innervation of the iliohypogastric and the ilioinguinal nerve. The anterior superior iliac spine and the pubic tubercle are marked as is the normal position for the incision for repair of inguinal hernia or orchidopexy

medial to the anterior superior iliac spine to finish its course running beneath the aponeurosis of the external oblique. It is possible, by depositing a large volume of bupivacaine beneath the external oblique aponeurosis one patient's fingerwidth medial to the anterior superior iliac spine, to block both these nerves. However, a number of failed blocks may occur if only this technique is used and it is better if a second injection is made medial to the anterior superior iliac spine to block the iliohypogastric nerve and the subcostal nerve if it is involved in the afferent pathways. These blocks are shown in detail in Fig. 4.13.

Many surgeons prefer to perform the operation of orchidopexy on young in-patients in the belief that a short period of bed-rest immediately following the procedure helps to prevent scrotal swelling. However, it is becoming more popular to carry out this procedure in selected patients on an out-patient basis. Although the upper wound for an orchidopexy is similar to that for repair of an inguinal hernia, a second wound is made in the scrotum when the testis is fixed in a dartos pouch. It may be that this incision is made in the area of the scrotum innervated by the ilioinguinal nerve. It is common for surgeons to extend this incision on to the inferior part of the scrotum which is innervated by the pudendal nerve. Pain arising from this area can be prevented if bupivacaine is infiltrated subcutaneously in the scrotum (Fig. 4.14), after the induction of anaesthesia along with the iliohypogastric and ilioinguinal nerve blocks, or

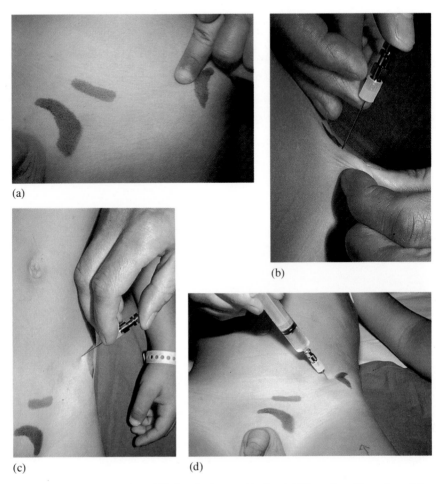

Fig. 4.13   Iliohypogastric and ilioinguinal nerve blocks. (a) The point of insertion of the needle is one of the patient's fingerbreadths medial to the anterior superior iliac spine. (b) The skin is picked up and a short bevelled, 22 gauge spinal needle is inserted through it so that its point comes to lie on the aponeurosis of the external oblique muscle. (c) The needle is *slowly* inserted and as it meets the resistance of the aponeurosis a large dimple in the skin begins to form. As the needle is further inserted the resistance of the aponeurosis becomes greater until with a sudden 'pop' the needle passes through the aponeurosis and, for a unilateral block, a half to a third of the syringe of local anaesthetic can be injected. (d) The needle point is gently withdrawn to its point of insertion and redirected downwards and slightly outwards. If this is done slowly the needle point can be felt passing through the external and internal oblique muscles until it strikes the inside of the ilium. A track of local anaesthetic can then be laid down as the needle is slowly withdrawn. Approximately a half to one third of the local anaesthetic should be used for a unilateral block

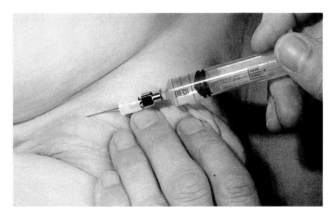

Fig. 4.14 Subcutaneous infiltration of the pudendal nerve innervation of the scrotum for orchidopexy. 1 ml of 0.5% bupivacaine can be injected subcutaneously in the inferior part of the scrotum and if squeezed it rapidly spreads in the lax subcutaneous tissue

intraoperatively by the surgeon after he has made his incision, 1 ml of 0.5% bupivacaine being sufficient.

A suitable dose of bupivacaine for these blocks would be in the order of 1 mg/kg for a unilateral block and 2 mg/kg for a bilateral block. Using such a regime, Epstein *et al.* (1988) found the C_{max} to be in the order of 1.35 μg/ml at T_{max} ranging from 10−40 minutes. This is much less than the plasma concentration generally thought to cause CNS toxicity in adults.

These blocks are generally safe and effective. Faulty technique, either due to depositing the local anaesthetic too close to the inguinal ligament (i.e. medial and *inferior* to the anterior superior iliac spine) or using an inappropriately large volume of local anaesthetic, can result in temporary femoral nerve block with paralysis of the quadriceps muscles. This can be troublesome and delay full ambulation of the patient. An explanation that it is of a temporary nature is normally all that is required to reassure patients and parents.

For circumcision

There has been more discussion of methods available to block pain following circumcision than any other paediatric surgical procedure possibly because of the frequency of performing this procedure and the assumption that it is an exceptionally painful procedure. Many authors suggest that the severe pain lasts only for the first two or three hours postoperatively and this could account for the success of Tree-Trakarn and Pirayavaraporn (1985) with topical lignocaine applied to the glans penis.

For many paediatric anaesthetists a block of the dorsal nerve of the penis or penile block is the first choice for preventing pain following circumcision.

Yoeman *et al.* (1983) and Vater and Wandless (1985) found this block to be superior to caudal extradural analgesia.

Brown *et al.* (1989) have described the anatomy of the dorsal nerve of the penis. It is a terminal branch of the pudendal nerve (S2, 3, and 4) which arises in the pudendal canal and runs forward along the ramus of the ilium and then along the margin of the inferior ramus of the pubis. After passing through the gap between the perineal membranes and the inferior pubic ligament, it enters a triangular shaped space where it is blocked during a penile nerve block. The boundaries of this space are the symphysis pubis above, the corpora cavernosa below and the membranous layer of superficial fascia anteriorly. The nerves lie on the dorsum of the penis lateral to the dorsal artery and vein, and give off a ventral branch early on their passage through the triangular shaped space which supplies the ventral surface of the penis including the frenulum. The suspensory ligament divides to form two sides of a triangle fusing with Buck's fascia which surrounds the penis and it is within the triangle formed by the division of the suspensory ligament that the dorsal nerves and their accompanying vessels lie.

Different modifications of blocks of the dorsal nerve of the penis have been described. Injections in the mid line of the penis have the potential risk of damaging the dorsal vein with either intravascular injections or haematoma formation. To avoid this, Soliman and Tremblay (1978) advocated a single shot lateral approach. This may not always provide adequate postoperative analgesia and bilateral blocks are more efficient (Fig. 4.15). The dose of local anaesthetic for this block is shown in Table 4.1. Bupivacaine 0.5% is the local anaesthetic of choice; *no vasoconstrictor should be used for this block*.

Of all the commonly performed peripheral nerve blocks this is the most difficult to master; the main problem is that of accurately estimating the depth of the needle before injecting the local anaesthetic. Morton *et al.* (1991) have drawn attention to this fact in the audit of anaesthetic practice in a busy paediatric day surgery unit, circumcision being the surgical procedure associated with most postoperative pain, i.e. the highest incidence of failed block. For this reason, some paediatric anaesthetists opt to use a caudal extradural block despite any reservations they might have about troublesome postoperative complications which can arise with this central block.

Table 4.1 Dosage of plain bupivacaine 0.5% for penile block

Age group (years)	Dose (ml)
Neonates	0.5
1	1.0
6	2.0
12	4.0

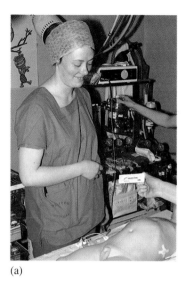

(a)

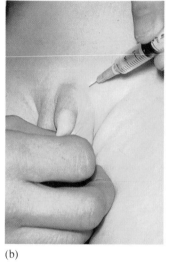

(b)

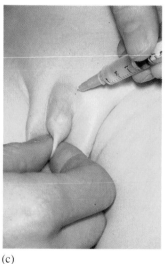

(c)

Fig. 4.15 Block of the dorsal nerve of the penis (Soliman and Tremblay 1978). (a) The anaesthetic nurse double checks that bupivacaine without adrenaline is being used. (b) A fine needle is inserted about the breadth of the patient's little finger lateral to the midline at '2 o'clock' to make contact with the symphysis pubis. (c) It is then passed deep to the symphysis pubis and slightly upwards towards the patient's head aiming for the centre of the imaginary clock face. A click may be felt as it passes through the superficial fascia. If there is any resistance to injection of the local anaesthetic at this point the needle should be slightly withdrawn. The block should then be repeated at '10 o'clock'. The dose of local anaesthetic for this block is shown in Table 1

For otoplasty

Although subcutaneous infiltration with bupivacaine can relieve the pain associated with otoplasty (Fig. 4.11), a block of the great auricular nerve is simple to perform and produces a duration of analgesia well in excess of that produced by infiltration. The great auricular nerve is a branch of the superficial cervical plexus and supplies all of the posterior surface of the ear and the lower two-thirds of the outer surface of the ear. It can be simply blocked as shown in Fig. 4.16. As subcutaneous infiltration with bupivacaine and adrenaline is an important method of providing haemostasis for this operation, it is not uncommon for a block of the great auricular nerve and infiltration to be carried out at the same time.

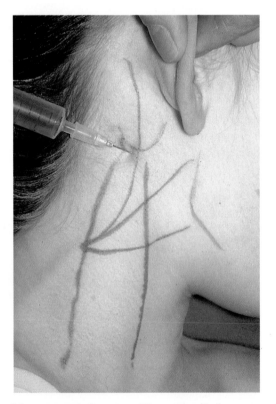

Fig. 4.16 Block of the great auricular nerve. The great auricular nerve, a branch of the superficial cervical plexus, becomes superficial at the midpoint of the posterior border of the sternomastoid muscle in the region of the external jugular vein. It can be blocked by injecting 3–4 ml of 0.5% bupivacaine with adrenaline subcutaneously from the mastoid process towards the descending ramus of the mandible

For orthopaedics

Many orthopaedic procedures of a minor nature are carried out on paediatric out-patients which are amenable to either simple techniques of local infiltration or distal peripheral nerve blockade. Release of trigger thumbs or fingers, excision of accessory digits, and tenotomies for curly toes are typical examples. Some children's digits are extremely small so ring block or digital block are best avoided as there is a real chance of end-artery damage if too large a volume of local anaesthetic is injected. However, more proximal blocks such as metacarpal and metatarsal blocks are alternatives which are easy to perform and effective (Figs 4.17, 4.18).

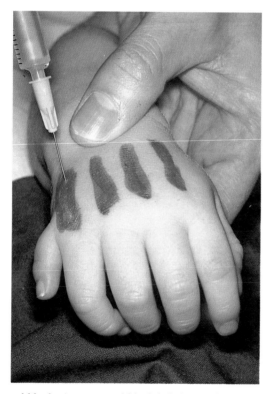

Fig. 4.17 Metacarpal block. A metacarpal block is being performed for excision of an accessory digit. A metacarpal block is performed by inserting the needle through the skin on the dorsum of the hand close to the base (proximal end) of the metacarpal until it is felt on the palm of the hand by the operator's left hand. Plain bupivacaine is injected until it is felt as a swelling on the palm and then the needle is slowly withdrawn as the local anaesthetic is injected. Depending on the site of surgery this can be repeated at various interspaces

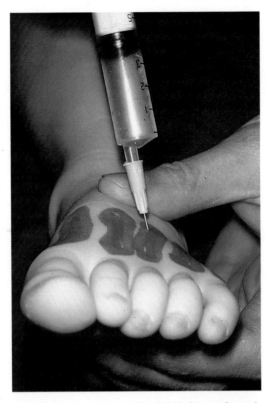

Fig. 4.18 Metatarsal block. A metatarsal block is being performed prior to correcting a curly middle toe. It is performed exactly like a metacarpal block, plain bupivacaine being injected at the proximal end of the metatarsal bone until a swelling is felt with the left hand on the sole of the foot. The needle is slowly withdrawn as the local anaesthetic continues to be injected. The needle should then be passed in to the adjacent interspace and the block repeated to ensure analgesia of the whole toe. If only two interspaces are involved then 0.5% bupivacaine can be used but for more widespread surgery involving multiple metatarsal blocks 0.25% plain hupivacaine should be used

Caudal extradural block

Extradural blocks especially caudal extradural block are commonly performed in paediatric practice and have much to commend them. Many paediatric day case surgical procedures are of a minor or superficial nature and it would seem more appropriate to use a peripheral nerve block rather than a central block in these situations. There is no doubt that caudal extradural anaesthesia results in a certain degree of postoperative morbidity. In the studies comparing the effect

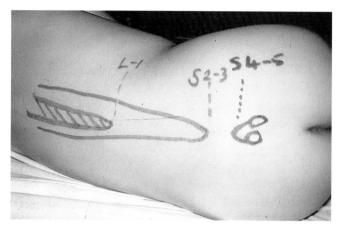

Fig. 4.19 Anatomy of the extradural space. The spinal cord (cross-hatched) can be seen ending at the lower border of the first lumber vertebra and the meninges in the region of the second or third sacral space. The sacral hiatus due to the unfused laminae of S4/5 is identified

of caudal anaesthesia and peripheral nerve blockade undesirable weakness of the legs and difficulty micturating have been found in the former group (Yoeman *et al.* 1983; Vater and Wandless 1985). Although these problems can be reduced by decreasing the concentration of local anaesthetic used they can not be eliminated, indeed nausea and vomiting associated with the use of caudal extradural anaesthesia may be as common or indeed worse than that found following the use of opioid analgesics (Lunn 1979; Bramwell *et al.* 1982; Martin 1982). This may be due to a rise in cerebrospinal fluid pressure.

The clinical significance of these complications is far from clear. In the UK not every child has the benefit of private transport home. If the ideal recovery from anaesthesia includes the ability to walk, micturate, and eat and drink liberally, then caudal extradural block may be associated with a delay in discharge or indeed may exclude discharge. Other disadvantages of caudal extradural block include potentially catastrophic complications such as inadvertent intravascular injection and subdural injection of local anaesthetic. Long-term complications such as haematoma and abscess formation also have to be considered. Despite these well documented complications some anaesthetists will still perform a caudal extradural block to prevent postoperative pain associated with circumcision and orchidopexy, especially if bilateral.

The anatomy of the extradural space is described in Fig. 4.19. The spinal cord reaches the third lumbar vertebra at birth and its relative position moves proximally over the first year of life until in adults and children over one year of age, it lies at the lower border of the first lumbar vertebra. The meninges reach the lower level of S2 or 3 at birth and remain there as the child grows. The sacral hiatus is at S4/5 and thus in very young children the distance from the sacral hiatus to the meninges is not great and there is a real risk of dural puncture if due care is not taken.

Although it is traditional to palpate the sacral cornua to find the sacral hiatus this, in practice, can often be difficult as the surface of the sacrum has many bumps which can be confused for these landmarks. Traditionally it is advised that once the cornua are identified a needle is inserted between them through skin, subcutaneous tissue, and the sacrococcygeal membrane. However, because of the unpredictability of finding the cornua this simple approach often fails. Therefore, once the cornua are thought to have been identified, feel for the sacrococcygeal membrane itself as a tight drumskin and only if this landmark is identified should a needle then be inserted through it (Figs 4.20–22).

A click can be felt as the needle passes through the sacrococcygeal membrane and to confirm that it is accurately placed the 'bounce test' should be performed. The syringe of local anaesthetic is attached firmly to the needle and the barrel depressed with frequent short sharp 'bounces'. If the barrel moves down the syringe with each 'bounce' and a small volume of local anaesthetic is injected then the needle is almost certainly correctly positioned. If the barrel moves back with each short sharp 'bounce' then it is almost certainly not in the extradural space. It should be possible to inject local anaesthetic into the extradural space with minimal resistance. Evidence of swelling would indicate that the needle was malpositioned in the subcutaneous tissue.

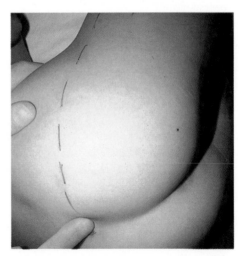

Fig. 4.20 Caudal extradural block—identification of the sacral hiatus. With the patient in the left lateral position and the legs placed at right angles to the trunk, the sacral hiatus can be identified by following a line drawn through the middle of the thighs which continues down across the buttocks

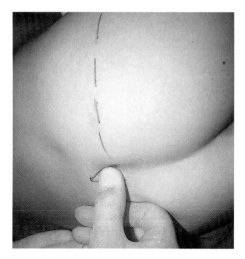

Fig. 4.21 Caudal extradural block—identification of the sacrococcygeal membrane. Identification of this membrane is crucial for the success of this block. Once the sacral cornua are believed to have been identified the sacrococcygeal membrane can be felt between them with the thumb as a tight drumskin. The needle should not be inserted until the sacrococcygeal membrane has been identified

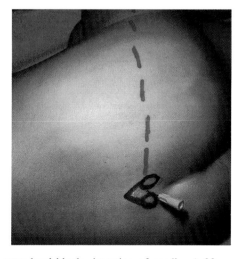

Fig. 4.22 Caudal extradural block—insertion of needle. A 23 gauge needle has been passed through skin, subcutaneous structures and the sacrococcygeal membrane during which a definite click can be felt. Note that once the needle has entered the extradural space there is no need to advance it proximally up the space as in small children the distance from the sacral hiatus to the meninges is not great and a dural tap is a real possibility

Table 4.2 Systemic analgesics for paediatric day cases

Indication	Drug	Dose (mg/kg)	Frequency	Route
Mild pain adjunct	Paracetamol	15–20 g	4 to 6 hourly	Oral, P.R.
Moderate pain adjunct	Diclofenac	1	6 hourly	P.R.
Pre-emptive analgesia	Ketorolac	0.5	6 hourly	IM, IV
Balanced analgesia	Ibuprofen	2.5–10	6 hourly	Oral
Break through pain	Dihydrocodeine	0.5	4 to 6 hourly	Oral
Failed local analgesia	Codeine	0.5 1	4 to 6 hourly 6 hourly	Oral IM, P.R.
	Morphine	1–0.2	3 to 6 hourly	IV, IM

For circumcision a volume of 0.3–0.4 ml/kg of 0.25% bupivacaine provides adequate analgesia with minimal motor weakness and 0.6–0.7 ml/kg is suitable for orchidopexy.

Conclusion

The intraoperative use of the long acting local anaesthetic agent bupivacaine can produce long lasting postoperative analgesia of high quality. Children rapidly recover from general anaesthesia, take food and drink at an early stage, are soon up and about, and discharged. This method of analgesia is only the beginning of the patient's postoperative analgesic requirements. Systemic analgesics (most commonly paracetamol) should be administered before any local anaesthetic block wears off (Table 4.2).

References

Arthur, D. S. and McNicol, L. R. (1986). Local anaesthetic techniques in paediatric surgery. *British Journal of Anaesthesia*, **58**, 760–78.

Badgwell, J. M., Heavner, J. E., and Kytta, J. (1990). Bupivacaine toxicity in young pigs is age dependent and is affected by volatile anaesthetics. *Anesthesiology*, **72**, 297–303.

Borgeat, A. and Wilder-Smith, O. (1991). Acute choreoathetoid reaction to propofol. *Anaesthesia*, **46**, 797.

Borgeat, A., Dessibourg, C., Popovic, V., Meier, D., Blanchard, M., and Schwander, D. (1991). Propofol and spontaneous movements: an EEG study. *Anesthesiology*, **74**, 24–7.

Bramwell, R. G. B., Bullen, C., and Radford, P. (1982). Caudal block for post-operative analgesia in children. *Anaesthesia*, **37**, 1024–6.

Brown, T. C. K., Weidner, N. J., and Bouwmeester, J. (1989). Dorsal nerve of penis block—anatomical and radiological studies. *Anaesthesia and Intensive Care*, **17**, 34–8.

Bush, G. H. and Roth, F. (1961). Muscle pains after suxamethonium in children. *British Journal of Anaesthesia*, **33**, 151–5.

Cameron, E., Johnston, G., Crofts, S., and Morton, N. S. (1992). Minimum effective dose of lignocaine to prevent injection pain due to propofol in children. *Anaesthesia*, **47**, 604–6.

Casey, W. F., Rice, L. J., Hannallah, R. S., Broadman, L., Norden, J. M., and Guzzetta, P. (1990). A comparison between bupivacaine instillation versus ilioinguinal/ iliohypogastric nerve block for post-operative analgesia following inguinal hernior-rhaphy in children. *Anesthesiology*, **72**, 637–9.

Cohen, M. M., Cameron, C. B., and Duncan, P. G. (1990). Paediatric anaesthesia morbidity and mortality in the perioperative period. *Anesthesia and Analgesia*, **70**, 160–7.

Coley, S. (1989). Anaesthesia of the skin. *British Journal of Anaesthesia*, **62**, 4–5.

Coté, C. J., Goudsouzian, N. G., Liu, L. M. P., Dedrick, D. F., and Rosow, C. E. (1981). The dose response of intravenous thiopental for induction of general anaesthesia in unpremedicated children. *Anesthesiology*, **55**, 703–5.

Doyle, E., McFadzean, W., and Morton, N. S. (1993). I. V. anaesthesia with propofol using a target-controlled infusion system: comparison with inhalation anaesthesia for general surgical procedures in children. *British Journal of Anaesthesia*, **70**, 542–5.

Epstein, R. H., Larijani, G. E., Wolfson, P. J., Ala-Kokko, T. I., and Boerner, T. F. (1988). Plasma bupivacaine concentrations following ilioinguinal/iliohypogastric nerve blockade in children. *Anesthesiology*, **69**, 773–6.

Fell, D., Derrington, M. C., Taylor, E., and Wandless, J. G. (1988). Paediatric post-operative analgesia. *Anaesthesia*, **43**, 107–10.

Freeman, J. A., Doyle, E., Ng, T. I., and Morton, N. S. (1993). Topical anaesthesia of the skin: a review. *Paediatric Anaesthesia*, **3**, 129–38.

Haynes, S. R. and Morton, N. S. (1993). The laryngeal mask airway: a review of its use in paediatric anaesthesia. *Paediatric Anaesthesia*, **3**, 65–73.

Lerman, J. (1992). Pharmacology of inhalational anesthetics in infants and children. *Paediatric Anaesthesia*, **2**, 191–203.

Lunn, J. N. (1979). Post-operative analgesia after circumcision. *Anaesthesia*, **34**, 552–4.

Lyle, D. J. R. (1982). Suxamethonium pains in outpatient children. *Anaesthesia*, **37**, 774–5.

McGinn, G., Haynes, S. R., and Morton, N. S. (1993). An evaluation of the laryngeal mask airway during routine paediatric anaesthesia. *Paediatric Anaesthesia*, **3**, 23–8.

McNicol, L. R. (1991). Insertion of laryngeal mask airway in children. *Anaesthesia*, **46**, 330.

Martin, L. V. H. (1982). Post-operative analgesia after circumcision in children. *British Journal of Anaesthesia*, **54**, 1263–6.

Mazoit, J. X., Denson, D. D., and Samii, K. (1988). Pharmacokinetics of bupivacaine following caudal anaesthesia in infants. *Anesthesiology*, **68**, 387–91.

Mirakhur, R. K. (1988). Induction characteristics of propofol in children: comparison with thiopentone. *Anaesthesia*, **43**, 593–8.

Mobley, K. A., Wandless, J. G., and Fell, D. (1991). Serum bupivacaine concentrations following wound infiltration in children undergoing inguinal herniotomy. *Anaesthesia*, **46**, 500–1.

Morton, N. S. (1990). Abolition of injection pain due to propofol in children. *Anaesthesia*, **45**, 70.

Morton, N. S., Wee, M., Christie, G., Gray, I. G., and Grant, I. S. (1988). Propofol for induction of anaesthesia in children. A comparison with thiopentone and halothane inhalational induction. *Anaesthesia*, **43**, 350–5.

Morton, N. S., Arthur, D. S., Cattanach, D., Fyfe, A., Best, C. J., and Haynes, K. A. (1991). Day case surgery for children. *Health Bulletin*, **49**, 54–61.

Morton, N. S., Johnston, G., White, M., and Marsh, B. J. (1992). Propofol in paediatric anaesthesia: a review. *Paediatric Anaesthesia*, **2**, 89–97.

Pandit, U. A., Stende, G. M., and Leach, A. B. (1985). Induction and recovery characteristics of isoflurane and halothane anaesthesia for short outpatient procedures in children. *Anaesthesia*, **40**, 1226–30.

Puttick, N. and Rosen, M. (1988). Propofol induction and maintenance with nitrous oxide in paediatric outpatient dental anaesthesia. *Anaesthesia*, **43**, 646–9.

Reid, M. F., Harris, R., Phillips, P. D., Barker, I., Pereira, N. H., and Bennett, N. R. (1987). Day care herniotomy in children. A comparison of ilioinguinal nerve block and wound infiltration for postoperative analgesia. *Anaesthesia*, **42**, 658–61.

Runcie, C. J., MacKenzie, S., Arthur, D. S., and Morton, N. S. (1993). Comparison of recovery from anaesthesia induced in children with either propofol or thiopentone. *British Journal of Anaesthesia*, **70**, 192–5.

Sampaio, M. M., Crean, P. M., Keilty, S. R., and Black, G. W. (1989). Changes in oxygen saturation during inhalational induction of anaesthesia in children. *British Journal of Anaesthesia*, **62**, 199–200.

Short, S. M. and Aun, C. S. T. (1991). Haemodynamic effects of propofol in children. *Anaesthesia*, **46**, 783–5.

Simmons, M., Miller, C. D., Cummings, G. C., and Todd, J. G. (1989). Outpatient paediatric dental anaesthesia. A comparison of halothane, enflurane and isoflurane. *Anaesthesia*, **44**, 735–8.

Soliman, M. G. and Tremblay, N. A. (1978). Nerve block of the penis for post-operative pain relief in children. *Anaesthesia and Analgesia*, **57**, 495.

Stokes, M. A. and Clutton-Brock, T. H. (1990). Monitoring infants and neonates. *Current Anaesthesia and Critical Care*, **1**, 147–53.

Stuart, J. C. and Morton, N. S. (1991). A clinical audit of day case surgery for children. *Journal of One Day Surgery*, **1**, 15–18.

Tree-Trakarn, T. and Pirayavaraporn, S. (1985). Post-operative pain relief for circumcision in children: comparison among morphine, nerve block and topical analgesia. *Anesthesiology*, **62**, 519–22.

Tucker, G. T. and Mather, L. E. (1979). Clinical pharmacokinetics of local anaesthetic agents. *Clinical Pharmacokinetics*, **4**, 241–78.

Tucker, G. T. and Mather, L. E. (1986). Pharmacokinetics of local anaesthetic agents. In *Neural blockade in clinical anaesthesia and management of pain*. (2nd edn) (ed. M. J. Cousins and P. O. Bridenbaugh), pp. 45–85. Lippincott, Philadelphia.

Vater, M. and Wandless, J. (1985). Caudal or dorsal nerve block? A comparison of two local anaesthetic techniques for post-operative analgesia following day case circumcision. *Acta Anaesthesiologica Scandinavica*, **29**, 175–9.

Watcha, M. F., Simeon, R. M., White, P. F., and Stevens, J. L. (1991). Effect of propofol on the incidence of postoperative vomiting after strabismus surgery in pediatric outpatients. *Anesthesiology*, **75**, 204–9.

Watson, D. M. (1991). Topical amethocaine in strabismus surgery. *Anaesthesia*, **46**, 368–70.

Yoeman, P. M., Cooke, R., and Hain, W. R. (1983). Penile block for circumcision. A comparison with caudal blockade. *Anaesthesia*, **38**, 862–6.

Zwass, M. S., Fisher, D. M., Welborn, L. G., Coté, C. J., Davis, P. J., Dinner, M., *et al.* (1992). Induction and maintenance characteristics of anaesthesia with desflurane and nitrous oxide in infants and children. *Anesthesiology*, **76**, 373–8.

5 Surgical techniques

P. A. M. Raine, A. H. B. Fyfe, A. A. F. Azmy, D. Attwood, N. K. Geddes, J. G. Boorman, G. C. Bennet, and J. Dudgeon

On the day of admission and immediately prior to the procedure, the surgeon or his nominated deputy must discharge a number of responsibilities made additionally important by the limited time available in the day case setting and the apparently simple and routine nature of much of the work.

Preoperative examination

The patient must be examined and the parents questioned carefully to establish that there has been no change in the surgical condition since the out-patient examination. Lesions may both resolve and progress in a short space of time. Hydroceles may disappear, a testis thought to have been arrested may have descended fully or a sebaceous cyst may have discharged.

Marking of side

The laterality of the lesion must be ascertained and noted (e.g. inguinal hernia, undescended testes, trigger thumb) and marked on the skin with indelible ink (Fig. 5.1).

Marking of site

The precise site of an abnormality should be marked on the skin (Fig. 5.2). A fatty epigastric hernia may be extremely difficult to palpate in the anaesthetized patient. Only one of a number of naevi may require excision.

Discussion of procedure

The exact nature of the procedure, site and size of the skin incision, and type of dressing should be discussed with the parent to prepare them for receiving the child postoperatively.

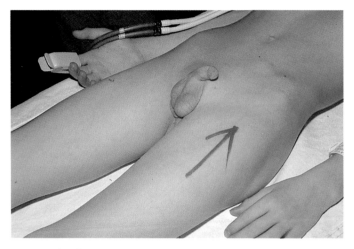

Fig. 5.1 Left side marked for inguinal herniotomy

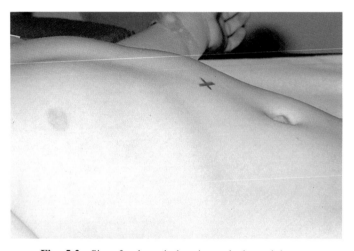

Fig. 5.2 Site of epigastric hernia marked on abdomen

Consent

Formal consent must be sought after the parent has been informed about the procedure. The parent may need help in following even a simple consent form in stressful preoperative circumstances. Published guidance on consent procedures should be followed (for example NHS in Scotland 1992).

In the induction room

It may be helpful for the surgeon to be present with the patient, parent, and anaesthetic team in the induction room. It offers an opportunity to examine again a previously fractious and difficult child immediately after induction. The most suitable position for the patient and the best line of access can be discussed (e.g. for excision of a lesion on the back of a patient). The position of the airway tube (Fig. 5.3) and monitoring equipment can be agreed.

A number of procedures may be performed in the induction room as soon as the patient has been anaesthetized, for example division of tongue-tie, retraction of foreskin and separation of adhesions, EUA anus, removal of sutures, and avulsion of toe nail.

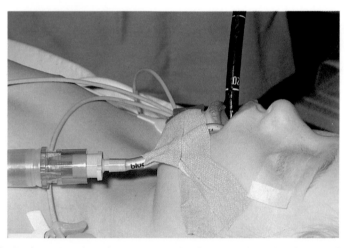

Fig. 5.3 Preformed endotracheal tube (south) fixed at left angle of mouth for upper gastrointestinal endoscopy

In the operating theatre

The operating theatre should have a system of identifying the precise requirements of each surgeon for a given procedure. Once the patient is anaesthetized time should not be wasted in acquiring unusual instruments or sutures. The surgeon is responsible for establishing preoperatively that his requirements will be met. Consideration should be given to:

(1) position of the patient on the operating table e.g. neck hyperextension to improve access (Fig. 5.4), armboard in place for hand surgery;

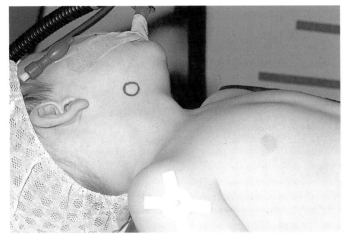

Fig. 5.4 Neck hyperextended to improve access to right cervical lump

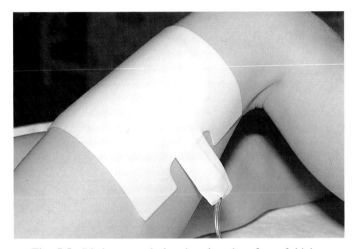

Fig. 5.5 Diathermy pad placed on broad surface of thigh

(2) use of diathermy. If it is to be used, the diathermy pad should be securely fixed to as broad and smooth a surface as possible (e.g. thigh or buttock) (Fig. 5.5);

(3) type of skin preparation (e.g. povidone iodine or chlorhexidine);

(4) arrangement of theatre lights (e.g. main light or satellite);

(5) use of magnification (e.g. microscope or loops).

General paediatric, urological, and plastic surgical procedures

Removal of skin and subcutaneous lesions

Small superficial operative procedures may be performed under either general or local anaesthesia. When local anaesthetic infiltration is used, adrenaline (1:200 000) may be added to produce haemostasis and improved visualization. Application of EMLA cream at the site of the lesion one and a half hours preoperatively will allow painless infiltration of local anaesthetic and adrenaline (see Chapter 4).

A number of important principles must be observed in excision of skin and subcutaneous lesions.

1. Incisions should be aligned in the skin tension lines.
2. Incisions across skin flexion lines must be avoided.
3. Per operative haemostasis must be secured—bipolar diathermy is suitable.
4. Dead space must be obliterated at the time of wound closure.
5. Fine suture techniques should be employed to produce minimal scarring.

Appropriate suture materials are: synthetic absorbable sutures in the subcuticular layer (which are best avoided on the face due to the slight risk of hypertrophy) and synthetic monofilament sutures which may be inserted as either interrupted suture or continuous subcuticular suture with a tie-over dressing (Fig. 5.6). Such sutures are easily removed and leave little mark on the skin.

Adhesive wound strips (Fig. 5.7) and tissue glue (Fig. 5.8) may also be used to coapt regular wounds and produce minimal scarring.

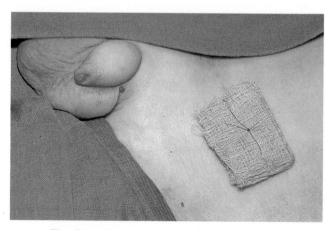

Fig. 5.6 'Tie-over' subcuticular nylon suture

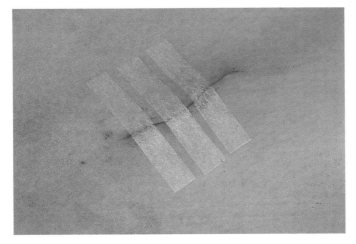

Fig. 5.7 Adhesive wound strips

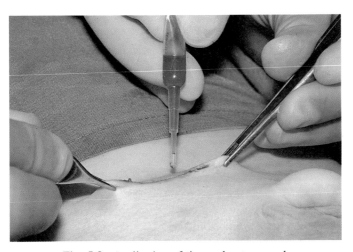

Fig. 5.8 Application of tissue glue to wound

External angular dermoid

An external angular dermoid is a congenital cystic swelling which may be noticed at birth or in the first few years of life. It is situated deep to the lateral aspect of the eyebrow (Fig. 5.9). If, due to its immobility, suspicion is raised that the cyst has an intracranial extension through a bony defect ('dumb-bell'), preoperative radiographs or CT scan should be obtained. Before surgery, local anaesthetic (containing 1:200 000 adrenaline) is infiltrated both to reduce

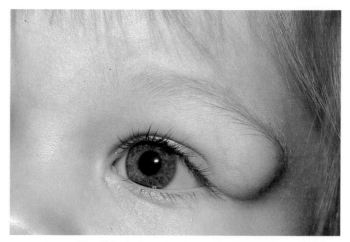

Fig. 5.9 Left external angular dermoid

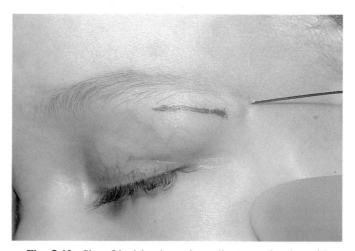

Fig. 5.10 Site of incision in eyebrow line to excise dermoid

bleeding perioperatively and to provide postoperative analgesia. An incision is made in the line of the eyebrow (Fig. 5.10) after shaving hair. In order to avoid transecting hair shafts, the incision is bevelled in the direction in which the hair shaft lie. Using skin hooks to retract the wound edges (Fig. 5.11), the incision is deepened until the cyst, usually creamy in colour, is identified. The surrounding tissues are then separated from the cyst by dissection with fine scissors. Many of these cysts are quite firmly attached to the underlying bone and the final

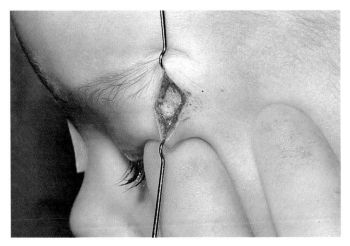

Fig. 5.11 Retraction of wound edges with skin hooks

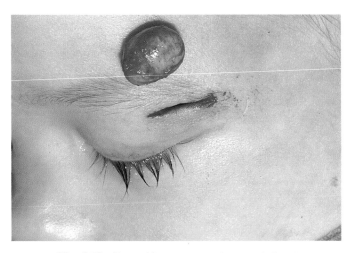

Fig. 5.12 Dermoid cyst removed: wound closed

removal can be effected with a small cleft palate rasp. In this way, the cyst can be removed intact and submitted for histological examination (Fig. 5.12).

Haemostasis is secured using bipolar diathermy. In closing the wound, it is important to eliminate the dead space created by the removal of the cyst with fine plain cat gut sutures. The skin incision may be closed either with fine interrupted sutures or a removable nylon subcuticular stitch. Sutures are removed after four to five days.

Preauricular skin tags

These common congenital anomalies (Fig. 5.13) may be seen in isolation or associated with other abnormalities of the face and ear. They present as variable sized swellings, most commonly in the preauricular area of the cheek or towards the angle of the mouth. Almost invariably, a cartilaginous component is present and should be removed. A fusiform excision is planned around the tag or tags usually in a vertical orientation. After incising along the marked lines, the incision is deepened towards the cartilaginous stalk which is traced and transected more deeply using fine scissors. The deep layers of the wound are closed with plain cat gut sutures and the skin with interrupted fine sutures or a removable subcuticular stitch.

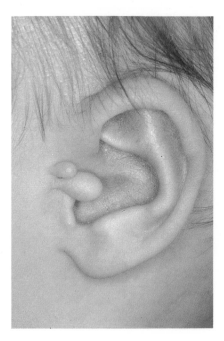

Fig. 5.13 Pre-auricular skin tags

Preauricular sinus

These small congenital sinuses are located at the junction of the upper end of the helix with the cheek. They are frequently asymptomatic but may be the site of infection with abscess formation. For this reason, their removal is usually recommended. Ink may be instilled into the sinus to make it easier to follow but the opening is frequently so narrow as to make this impracticable. A fusiform excision is made around the sinus opening and the tract is followed deeply using fine scissor dissection. It is frequently longer than expected and ends deeply against the cartilage. The wound is closed with fine interrupted sutures.

Removal of naevi and other cutaneous lesions

Cutaneous naevi are almost invariably benign in childhood (Fig. 5.14). However, if removal is advocated, this should include a small margin of 1−2 mm normal skin around the lesion. The excision should be designed so that the resulting scar lies in the relaxed skin tension lines to obtain an optimum result. In general, such lines are at right angles to the line of the underlying muscle pull and are approximately transverse on the limbs and trunk.

For smaller wounds, particularly on the face, interrupted fine monofilament sutures are appropriate, whilst for larger lesions and especially those on the trunk or limbs, a subcuticular absorbable stitch has advantages in providing longer wound support and minimizing scar stretching. It also avoids the necessity for suture removal which is appreciated by both the patient and the nursing staff. Following removal of a large lesion, the healing wound may be supported with adhesive wound strips and bandaging may be appropriate to reduce movement of adjacent joints for ten days to allow optimal wound healing.

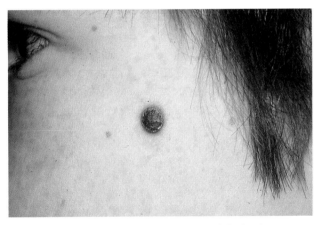

Fig. 5.14 Pigmented naevus on left cheek

Spider naevi

Spider naevi arise on the face (Fig. 5.15), nose, and malar areas in particular. They are small vascular lesions fed by a central arteriole whose ablation removes the associated blush. If local anaesthesia is used, adrenaline should not

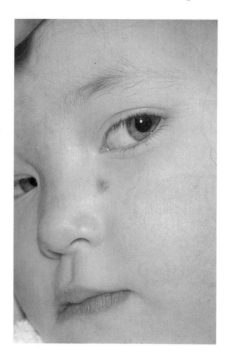

Fig. 5.15 Spider naevus

be incorporated as it may cause constriction of the feeding arteriole making the lesion difficult to see. Methods of ablation include:

(1) unipolar fine point diathermy;

(2) tunable dye laser.

The former is most often used but achieves only 70 per cent success at the first procedure. An alternative is to use a fine intravenous cannula whose plastic sheath provides some insulation for surrounding dermis and minimizes dermal scarring. The diathermy current is applied to the needle of the cannula once it has been located in the arteriole.

Prominent ears (bat ears)

Prominent ears are usually due to incomplete formation of the antehelical fold (Fig. 5.16) and can be readily corrected by a simple otoplasty involving creation of this fold. The procedure is amenable to day surgery though postoperative vomiting and discomfort may occur. More complex ear anomalies are better managed as in-patient procedures. Otoplasty is performed by excising a strip of skin on the posterior aspect of the pinna after first marking with indelible ink (methylene blue) the proposed position of the antehelical fold. The cartilage is

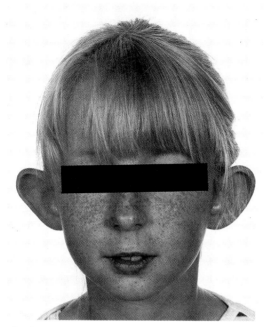

Fig. 5.16 Prominent (bat) ears with absent antehelical fold

folded appropriately and retained in its new position by non-absorbable mattress sutures. Methods of incising and scoring the cartilage also achieve this. The skin wound is closed using a continuous monofilament removable suture. Dressings are placed to conform to and support the ear shape and a head bandage is secured for ten days.

Lymph node biopsy

Lymph nodes in the neck, axilla, or groin may require excision biopsy for diagnostic or cosmetic reasons. The position of the patient is important to give good access; for neck glands the neck is extended and rotated and for axillary glands the arm is abducted. Skin incisions may include an ellipse if there is evidence of attachment to the skin and should be placed in skin tension lines. Nodes should be completely removed unless multiple or matted. A plane of dissection close to the gland should be followed and feeding vessels coagulated with diathermy. Residual dead space must be closed. Frozen section, formalin-fixed, saline, or dry specimens are submitted for histology, electron microscopy, or bacteriology as appropriate. It is advisable to contact the laboratory in advance of the procedure to establish how the specimen should be presented.

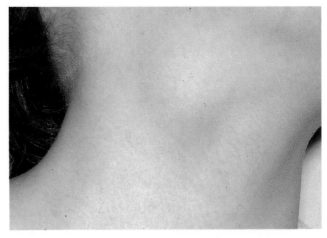

Fig. 5.17   Right tonsillar lymph gland enlargement due to atypical mycobacterium

Atypical mycobacterium characteristically causes enlargement of the tonsillar nodes (Fig. 5.17) with a normal chest X-ray and Mantoux test. Anti-tuberculous therapy is ineffective and complete excision is curative.

Other neck lumps

A variety of small neck lumps may be regarded as suitable for excision on a day basis. However, if deeper or more extensive dissection is likely to result in postoperative oedema sufficient to cause a degree of airway obstruction, in-patient observation will be needed. Thyroglossal and branchial cysts (Fig. 5.18) may be associated with tracts requiring such dissection. None the less, large series of paediatric day cases include branchial cleft anomalies and salivary gland lesions (Moir *et al.* 1987). Dermoid cysts, small haemangiomas and lymphangiomas, and ectopic salivary adenomas (Fig. 5.19) may be removed simply and safely as day procedures.

Inguinal hernia

Indirect inguinal hernia is a common occurrence in boys due to failure of complete obliteration of the *processus vaginalis*. Many present in the neonatal period or early infancy when problems of irreducibility and strangulation are potentially more serious—closure is a matter of relative urgency in infants under six months of age. In older infants and young boys these risks are less. Inguinal herniae occur more often on the right side than the left (8:1) and less often in

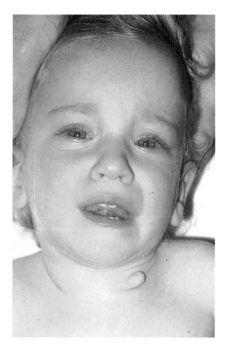

Fig. 5.18 Left branchial remnant (skin tag with cartilage) overlying branchial cyst

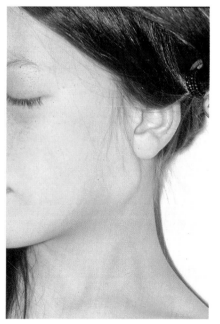

Fig. 5.19 Left submandibular salivary gland adenoma

girls (M:F, 5:1). The presence of a palpable gonad in an inguinal hernial sac in a girl raises the possibility of testicular feminizing syndrome; the nature of the gonad must be ascertained.

Most inguinal herniae can be satisfactorily dealt with on a day basis. In a very large series of over 10 000 cases, the complication rate was 0.84 per cent and only 0.12 per cent required in-patient admission after surgery (Yang 1991). Wound infection rates may be negligible (Mejdahl and Gyrtrup 1989). Large irreducible bilateral herniae may be better managed as in-patients due to the length of the procedure and the extent of dissection. Premature infants are usually dealt with as in-patients though day case series have been reported with satisfactory results (Melone *et al.* 1992).

Supplementation of general anaesthesia with a local anaesthetic technique such as caudal anaesthesia, ilioinguinal block, or wound infiltration with bupivacaine are used (see Chapter 4). The patient lies supine and the groin and perineal areas are prepared. A short incision is made in the inguinal skin crease just above the pubic ramus. This is deepened with diathermy and the subcutaneous fascia is

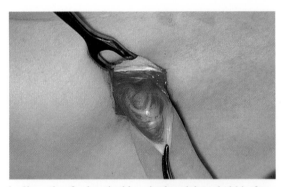

Fig. 5.20   Groin dissection for inguinal hernia; hernial sac held in forceps, vas also seen

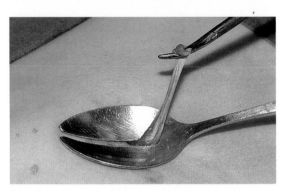

Fig. 5.21   Inguinal hernial sac dissected to its neck; vas and vessels retracted by slit spoon prior to transfixion ligation of sac

divided in the line of the wound. The superficial inferior epigastric vein is retracted or cauterized. The wound is retracted with skin hooks and the external oblique fascia is exposed just above the external inguinal ring. The fibres may be split down to the external ring or the hernial sac may be approached by division of the layers of spermatic fascia at the external ring. The ilioinguinal nerve is exposed and preserved. The sac is then delivered and carefully separated from vas and vessels (Fig. 5.20) which may be left undisturbed in the inguinal canal. The inguinal hernial sac is then cleared to its neck at the internal ring (Fig. 5.21) and transfixion ligated with 3/0 synthetic absorbable or black silk suture. If the testis has been displaced from the scrotum, it should be carefully replaced. The external oblique fascia is then repaired with 3/0 synthetic absorbable suture (Fig. 5.22) and the external inguinal ring tightened around the cord: it may be closed off completely in the female. The wound is closed with 3/0 absorbable sutures to the superficial fascia and subcutaneous tissues and 4/0 or 5/0 continuous subcuticular sutures (Fig. 5.23). An occlusive dressing is applied.

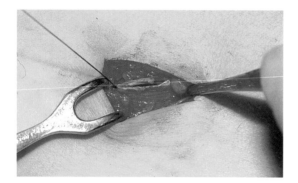

Fig. 5.22 Closure of external oblique fascia after herniotomy

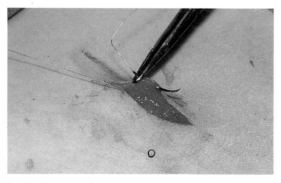

Fig. 5.23 Subcuticular continuous 5/0 absorbable suture

Hydrocele

Hydrocele occurs principally as a congenital anomaly due to incomplete obliteration of the *processus vaginalis* in communicating, non-communicating, and encysted forms. In girls, the hydrocele occurs in the canal of Nuck. The possibility of hydroceles secondary to infection, trauma, torsion, or tumour should be considered if the history is of recent or sudden onset or if the testis does not feel normal. In these cases, in-patient admission may be considered as inspection and, if necessary, biopsy of the testis is performed.

Spontaneous resolution of a communicating hydrocele may occur up to the age of four years and surgery is therefore usually delayed to this age. Encysted and non-communicating hydroceles persist. The indications for surgery are cosmetic appearance, discomfort, and occasionally interference with application of nappies and the early stages of walking (Fig. 5.24). The requirement for surgery is about one fifth that for inguinal herniotomy and hydroceles are approximately equally distributed between right and left.

The surgical procedure and technique is effectively the same as for inguinal herniotomy. The processus is ligated and hydrocele fluid is drained but no attempt is made to remove the hydrocele sac. Fluid may reaccumulate transiently.

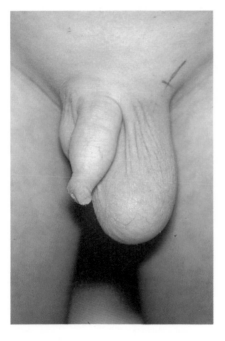

Fig. 5.24 Large communicating hydrocele

Orchidopexy

Undescended testis occurs slightly more commonly on the left than the right and has an incidence of 1.58 per cent at age three months (John Radcliffe Hospital Cryptorchidism Study Group 1986). Many authorities now consider that orchidopexy should be performed at around two years of age and that subsequent delay may lead to decreased fertility. Unequivocal evidence for this is scarce and orchidopexy before school age is often accepted as a satisfactory clinical compromise. Certain differentiation of ectopia or incomplete descent from retractile testis cannot always be made at the first presentation. The common site for ectopia is the superficial inguinal pouch; occasionally a testis is found in the thigh, perineum, or at the base of the penis. A testis may also be palpated at the neck of the scrotum or external inguinal ring in the line of normal descent. The procedure of orchidopexy is relatively straight forward in these cases and day surgery is appropriate.

In the more unusual circumstances in which the testis is impalpable, the possibilities are that it is intracanalicular, abdominal, or absent. In these circumstances, exploration and more extensive mobilization are needed. Day case surgery may not be appropriate in view of the length of procedure, the need for more prolonged anaesthesia and the requirement for postoperative immobilization and rest. Careful preoperative case selection and accurate assessment of the position of the testis is the key to a successful programme of day surgery. Over 90 per cent of orchidopexies have been performed as day cases with very low complication and high success rates (Gyrtrup et al. 1989).

Following general anaesthesia either caudal or ilioinguinal/iliohypogastric nerve block is used to relieve postoperative pain (see Chapter 4). The patient is placed in a supine position and the groin and the perineal areas are prepared. An inguinal crease incision is made (Fig. 5.25) and deepened with diathermy through the superficial fascia to expose the external oblique fascia above the external inguinal ring. The fascia is then split in the line of its fibres to open the inguinal canal and external inguinal ring. The testis is identified and mobilized with separation of the investing layers of spermatic fascia. The vas and vessels are carefully dissected from the inguinal hernial sac or processus. The sac is ligated and the vas and vessels further mobilized to the deep inguinal ring (Fig. 5.26) to give sufficient mobility to allow the testis to be placed at the bottom of the scrotum without tension. Occasionally this can be more readily achieved by re-routing the testis and cord medial to the deep inferior epigastric vessels at the medial aspect of the deep inguinal ring. Through a small scrotal skin incision, a subdartos pouch is fashioned between skin and dartos fascia in the lower part of the scrotum (Fig. 5.27). Forceps are then passed through the scrotal skin incision via a small defect in the dartos fascia up through the neck of the scrotum to grasp the testis in the inguinal wound. The testis is then drawn down into the subdartos pouch where it is retained.

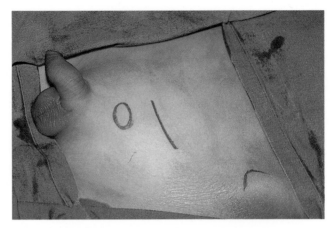

Fig. 5.25 Site of inguinal skin crease incision for orchidopexy (position of testis and superior anterior iliac spine also marked)

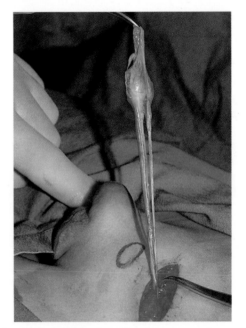

Fig. 5.26 Mobilization of testis on vas and vessels

The scrotal skin is then closed with 4/0 interrupted plain cat gut and further infiltrated with local anaesthetic as the ilioinguinal nerve block does not cover the lower scrotum. The inguinal wound is closed in layers with absorbable synthetic sutures.

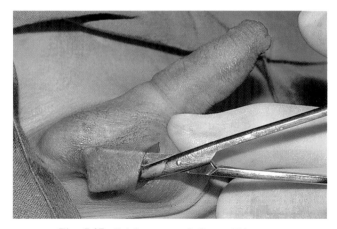

Fig. 5.27   Subdartos pouch for orchidopexy

Epigastric hernia

An epigastric hernia arises in the midline due to protrusion of extra peritoneal fat through a small defect in the *linea alba* (Fig. 5.28). It is commonly at about the mid-point between xiphisternum and umbilicus but may occur anywhere on this line. It is imperative that the site is accurately marked preoperatively (helped by the child standing) as the small hernia (usually less than 1 cm in diameter) may be extremely difficult to palpate in the relaxed anaesthetized patient.

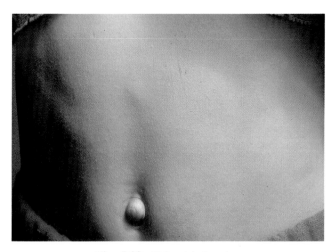

Fig. 5.28   Epigastric hernia

Occasionally, there is more than one defect. A short transverse skin incision is made and the herniated fat lump defined—it is usually easily differentiated from surrounding subcutaneous fat. The fascial defect may be only a few millimetres in diameter and may need to be extended to allow reduction of the hernia. The defect is then closed with synthetic absorbable interrupted sutures and the skin with a subcuticular suture.

Umbilical hernia

Between the sixth and tenth weeks of intrauterine life the mid-gut is partially extra-coelomic in the body stalk. An umbilical hernia is an outpouching of peritoneum through an incompletely obliterated umbilical ring following return of the extra-coelomic intestine into the abdominal cavity. It is common with an incidence of 4 per cent at six weeks of age and approximately 2 per cent at one year. Even large hernias in the young infant (Fig. 5.29) may spontaneously resolve with gradual closure of the umbilical ring and it is reasonable to wait until the child is four years old to allow this possibility. The hernia is rarely the cause of symptoms; though it may bulge alarmingly on crying, and obstruction or strangulation are extreme rarities. Repair is performed through a sub-umbilical incision made by an initial short midline stab split further laterally by opening forceps in a vertical plane to produce a symmetrical curved (lunar) incision (Fig. 5.30a. and b.). The neck of the hernial sac is surrounded by dissection and defined to the level of the fascia. The sac is opened and any

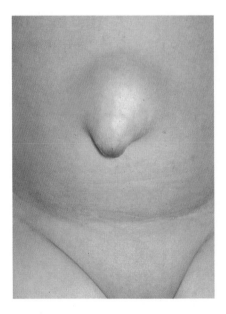

Fig. 5.29   Large umbilical hernia

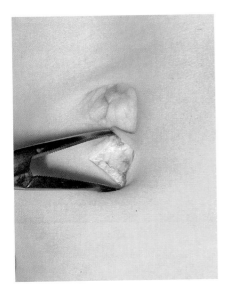

Fig. 5.30a Splitting subumbilical skin stab incision with forceps

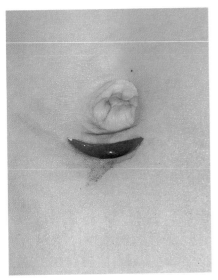

Fig. 5.30b Subumbilical lunar incision for umbilical hernia repair

omental or vitelline attachment must be carefully separated to avoid bleeding or obstruction. The neck of the sac is then closed flush with the midline fascia using interrupted sutures. The subumbilical incision lies in apposition and requires only a subcuticular suture or wound strips for closure.

Infiltration with bupivacaine is recommended at the beginning or the end of the procedure for postoperative analgesia (see Chapter 4).

Supra-umbilical hernia

This hernia occurs through a small defect just above the umbilical ring and does not therefore have any tendency to spontaneous obliteration. It is dealt with as for an epigastric hernia.

Circumcision

Circumcision is one of the commonest operations performed as a day case (Williams *et al.* 1993). Most are infants and young boys but occasionally an older boy may present with a scarred or non-retractile foreskin. The main indications for circumcision are:

(1) phimosis (constriction of the preputial orifice)—usually secondary to balanitis and scarring of the foreskin leading to non-retractibility. Congenital phimosis is a rare indication for circumcision;

(2) recurrent balanitis/posthitis;

(3) long, non-retractile foreskin in the older boy (over five years);

(4) paraphimosis.

A penile or caudal block provides regional anaesthesia. The boy is positioned supine with legs slightly separated. The penoscrotal area and suprapubic region is thoroughly prepared.

The foreskin is stretched using sinus forceps and completely retracted to expose the glans which is thoroughly cleaned. Retained smegma is removed. The foreskin is returned over the glans and held by tissue forceps. Sinus forceps are applied to mark the site of the proposed circumcision and to ensure that the glans is pushed proximally to avoid injury (Fig. 5.31). The foreskin is cleanly cut close to the sinus forceps using a blade or scissors. The forceps are removed and the outer layer of skin is retracted over the shaft of the penis to reveal subcutaneous bleeding points. The dorsal and two lateral veins of the penis and the frenular artery should be identified and ligated with cat gut. Other minor bleeding points should be similarly secured to ensure complete haemostasis. The urethral meatus is inspected for evidence of stenosis. Meatotomy is very occasionally required.

The deep mucosal layer of the foreskin is then excised circumferentially (starting from the frenulum) using forceps and curved scissors leaving a cuff of about 2 mm. Further bleeding may occur and should be secured. Mucosa and skin are then apposed with 4/0 plain cat gut interrupted sutures. Two corner stitches (ventral and dorsal) are initially inserted and held on traction to

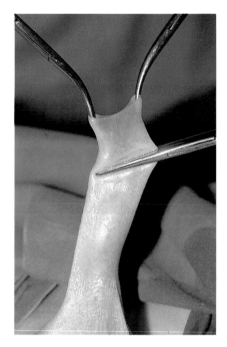

Fig. 5.31 Straight forceps applied to foreskin for circumcision

facilitate this (Fig. 5.32). At the frenulum, an 8-type stitch may be used for good approximation of the skin and to secure the frenular artery. After suturing, assessment of the final appearance should be made (Fig. 5.33). Occasionally redundant skin may need to be trimmed. Any ooze from the suture line requires an extra stitch.

The wound should be cleaned with cetrimide and a wrap-round dressing of soft paraffin gauze and light gauze may be applied to allow micturition. In addition to a penile or caudal block, lignocaine gel, ointment, or spray, may be applied around the glans (see Chapter 4). The dressing is normally removed by soaking in the bath on the following day.

Circumcision in the older child

In the older child, in order to achieve satisfactory cosmetic appearance and haemostasis, the preferred method of circumcision is by dissection. After cleaning, stretching, and retracting the foreskin, it is held by two mosquito forceps on the dorsal and ventral aspects. The foreskin is divided in the dorsal midline using scissors to the coronal sulcus; it is then trimmed around the coronal sulcus to the frenulum. The frenular artery is ligated and the skin completely excised. The lateral penile veins are defined and ligated and skin is apposed to mucosa with 4/0 plain cat gut.

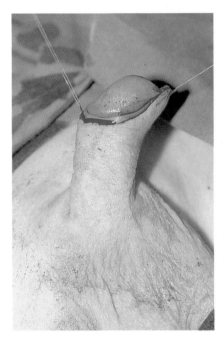

Fig. 5.32 Circumcision repair—corner stitches inserted

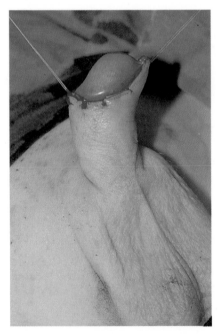

Fig. 5.33 Skin to mucosa suture of circumcision

Complications after circumcision

The principal complication is bleeding; either a slow ooze from the suture line or a brisk reactionary bleed into the dressings or into the penile tissues causing a haematoma of the penile shaft and scrotum.

Compression may control bleeding but further anaesthesia may be necessary to define and ligate the bleeding vessel. Haematoma may lead to prolonged pain and dysuria if bleeding is not controlled. Significant blood loss and shock may occur.

Injury to the glans or meatus is unusual but may occur if the foreskin is not fully separated from the glans at commencement. Bleeding will require attention and an attempt should be made to repair the glans without causing meatal stenosis.

Foreskin retraction and separation of preputial adhesions

Many cases of recurrent balanitis, discomfort on micturition, or ballooning of the foreskin are related to incomplete separation of foreskin from glans rather than to phimosis. Symptoms can be relieved by separation of preputial adhesions and retraction of the foreskin and circumcision is often unnecessary (Cooper *et al.* 1983, Gordon and Collin 1993). Suitability for retraction alone can be assessed by lifting the foreskin away from the glans and demonstrating that the preputial orifice is not constricted (Fig. 5.34).

Separation of foreskin is achieved by gentle retraction using gauze swabs (Fig. 5.35) or by sweeping a probe round the sub-preputial space. Smegma

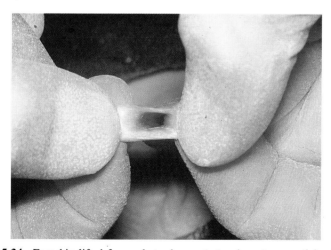

Fig. 5.34 Foreskin lifted forwards to demonstrate adequate preputial orifice

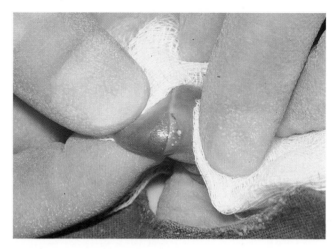

Fig. 5.35 Separation of foreskin/glans adhesions with gauze swab

may be released. Forcible stretching of the foreskin should be avoided as this will lead to fissuring, fibrosis, and phimosis. If the foreskin proves too tight to retract, circumcision should be performed.

After retraction of the foreskin, the glans is cleaned with cetrimide and soft paraffin is applied. The foreskin must be drawn down over the glans to its original position to avoid risks of paraphimosis. Postoperatively, the boy is encouraged to draw the foreskin back whilst bathing, wash beneath it, and apply soft paraffin daily—he may need the help of parents.

Meatal stenosis

Narrowing and stenosis of the external urinary meatus may be congenital, a result of recurrent balanoposthitis or a complication of previous circumcision. Examination usually reveals a shelf of glandular tissue encroaching on the meatus. This may be associated with a minor degree of glandular hypospadias.

Dorsal meatotomy or Y−V plasty

Dorsal meatotomy is performed by applying straight artery forceps to crush the shelf of tissue followed by division with straight scissors. The procedure is usually bloodless and no suturing or dressings are required. Occasionally it is more appropriate to perform meatotomy ventrally.

Y−V plasty is required for more marked meatal stenosis. A Y-incision is made using a size 11 blade across the dorsal rim of the urethral meatus which is widened by conversion to a V-closure using interrupted 5/0 chromic cat gut or synthetic absorbable suture.

Minor degrees of glandular and coronal sulcus hypospadias

Minor degrees of glandular and coronal sulcus hypospadias (Fig. 5.36) may be corrected by a meatal advancement and glanduloplasty procedure (MAGPI).

A stay stitch of 3/0 black silk is inserted in the glans with a round bodied needle and help by artery forceps. The urethral meatus is assessed for the suitability of this procedure and the presence of skin chordee is noted. Size 6 or 8 feeding tube is inserted per urethram into the bladder. A vertical incision is made into the substance of the glans from the dorsal margin of the meatus to the tip of the glans using a size 11 blade. To minimize bleeding a tourniquet is used. The meatus is advanced towards the tip of the glans by closing this incision transversely with four or five 5/0 synthetic absorbable interrupted sutures.

A transverse incision is made in the skin immediately proximal to the meatus and carried laterally into the coronal sulcus and circumferentially to the dorsum as a circumcision to divide completely the inner layer of foreskin from glans. The skin of the penile shaft is then dissected to release skin chordee. A traction suture is inserted at the ventral rim of the meatus and drawn distally allowing the wings of the glans to be apposed and sutured with interrupted 5/0 absorbable mattress sutures ventral to the meatus (Fig. 5.37). Excessive apposition will result in a conical appearance of the glans. The dorsal foreskin may be split vertically and used (as Byars flaps) to elongate the ventral penile surface. Excess

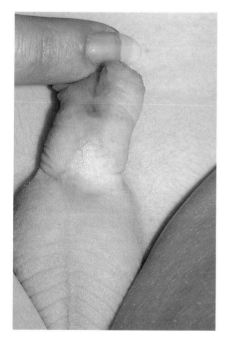

Fig. 5.36 Coronal hypospadias

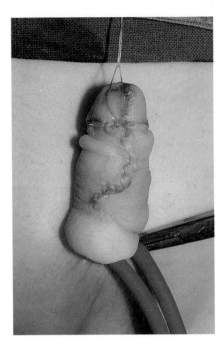

Fig. 5.37 MAGPI repair of hypospadias

foreskin is excised and careful skin to mucosa repair is performed at the coronal sulcus with 5/0 absorbable interrupted sutures.

At the conclusion, the tourniquet is released, the catheter is removed, and a firm dressing of sofratulle and gauze is applied. The dressing is usually kept in place for 24 hours and removed in the bath.

Minor revisions after repair of hypospadias

Minor procedures may be required to trim excess skin or perform a meatotomy following hypospadias repair. It is important to mark proposed incisions carefully with indelible ink to avoid inadequate or over-enthusiastic excision. Haemostasis must be secured and skin is closed with 5/0 absorbable interrupted sutures.

Correction of penoscrotal web

Penoscrotal web (Fig. 5.38) is an uncommon anomaly due to maldevelopment of the skin of the penoscrotal junction. It does not usually cause functional problems and correction is therefore performed for cosmetic reasons. The web may be incised transversely to produce a diamond-shaped defect which is closed longitudinally or a V–Y plasty may be performed to lengthen the raphe.

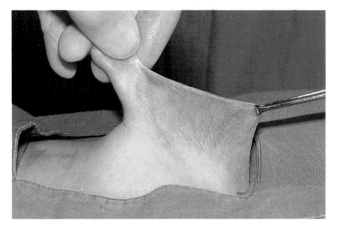

Fig. 5.38 Penoscrotal skin web

Interrupted 5/0 synthetic absorbable or cat gut sutures may be used. Dressings are not required.

Cystoscopy

The indications for cystourethroscopy in children are:

(1) haematuria;
(2) obstructive uropathy (e.g. urethral valves, neurogenic bladder, ureterocele);
(3) vesico-ureteric reflux;
(4) retrograde ureteric catheterization.

Cystoscopy in a small child is performed with the child lying supine with hips abducted, knees flexed, and feet taped together. Older children can be placed in the lithotomy position. If necessary, urethral dilatation is performed after preparation of the perineal area.

The cystoscope is passed gently into the bladder, which is thoroughly inspected taking particular note of the trigone and ureteric orifices (site, shape, and size are important). The possibility of duplex ureteric orifices is checked. The bladder neck and the whole length of urethra are inspected.

Vesico-ureteric reflux

Vesico-ureteric reflux may cause renal scarring early in life and subsequent long-term renal damage. There is a 4:1 female preponderance. Surgical intervention is indicated for:

(1) recurrent breakthrough infections;

(2) poor compliance with medical treatment;
(3) progressive or new renal scarring as determined by DMSA scan;
(4) duplex, refluxing ureters.

The 'Sting' procedure ('subureteric *teflon* *in*jection')

The 'Sting' technique (O'Donnell and Puri 1984) may be performed on a day case basis. It involves injecting per-cystoscope a small amount of Teflon paste submucosally at the vesico-ureteric junction. This creates a mound which converts the rounded ureteric orifice into a crescent shape (Fig. 5.39a. and b.). An 11.5 F.G. Wolff Sting Scope with angled eye-piece is used (Fig. 5.40). 89 per cent of refluxing ureters are successfully treated on the first injection (Fyfe and Azmy 1992); the remaining ureters require two or three injections to abolish reflux.

Following the procedure, the child can be discharged once he has passed urine. Prophylactic antibiotic therapy is continued and follow-up isotope scans are necessary to ensure that reflux has been abolished and that the ureter is not obstructed. Long-term follow-up to monitor renal growth is also important.

Recently, doubts have been raised about the safety of Teflon paste and the possibility of migration of particles. An alternative, 'Macroplastique', is currently in use as migration of particles appears less likely.

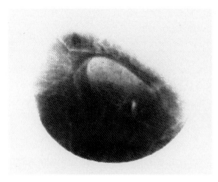

Fig. 5.39a Gaping ureteric orifice in vesico-ureteric reflux

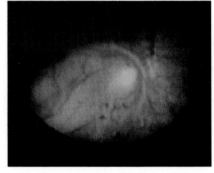

Fig. 5.39b Crescent shaped ureteric orifice after 'Sting' procedure

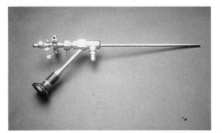

Fig. 5.40 Wolff 'Sting' cystoscope

Upper gastrointestinal endoscopy

Upper gastrointestinal endoscopy using either flexible or rigid instruments may be performed as a day procedure under sedation or general anaesthesia. No preparation other than preoperative fasting is necessary. Indications for upper gastrointestinal endoscopy include:

(1) recurrent epigastric pain;
(2) haematemesis;
(3) peptic ulcer disease;
(4) portal hypertension;
(5) gastro-oesophageal reflux;
(6) inflammatory bowel disease.

Good understanding and co-operation between endoscopist and anaesthetist is never more essential than when the airway is 'shared' (Fig. 5.41). A full endoscopic examination includes inspection and assessment of the oesophagus, cardia, stomach, antrum, pylorus, and first and second parts of the duodenum (Fig. 5.42). Video recording is helpful both at the time and for subsequent recall and analysis. Biopsy specimens may be needed for histological and micro-biological examination. Bleeding following biopsy is rare but, if suspected, a nasogastric tube should be inserted at the conclusion of the procedure. Oesophageal varices are not normally injected as a day case procedure due to the increased risk of early postoperative bleeding. At the conclusion of endoscopic examination the stomach should be sucked out to evacuate air and fluid and minimize the risk of postoperative vomiting.

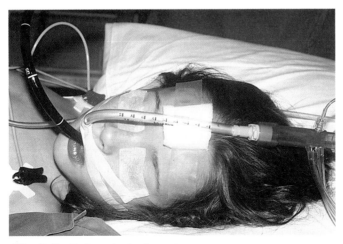

Fig. 5.41 Endotracheal tube and gastroscope—'shared' airway

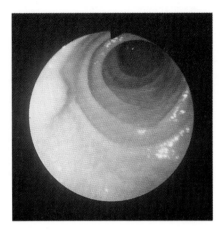

Fig. 5.42 Normal duodenal mucosal appearance at endoscopy

Lower gastrointestinal tract

Examination under anaesthetic, endoscopy, and biopsy of the perineum, anus, and rectum may be indicated in the investigation of constipation, painful defaecation, and bleeding per rectum. It may also be necessary in the documentation of known or suspected:

(1) polyposis;
(2) inflammatory bowel disease;
(3) anorectal anomaly;
(4) rectal or mucosal prolapse;
(5) child sexual abuse.

Examination

The examination is best performed with the patient lying either in the left lateral position with the right hip and knee flexed or supine with both hips and knees flexed. Important observations include:

(1) condition of the perianal skin—inflammation or bruising, perianal warts;
(2) the position of the anus—ectopic (anterior);
(3) patulous or stenotic anus;
(4) perianal skin tags or fissures (Fig. 5.43);
(5) evidence of mucosal or rectal wall prolapse.

Gentle eversion of the anal mucosa reveals the presence of a fissure—most commonly in the posterior position.

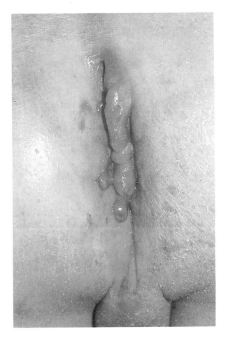

Fig. 5.43 Perianal skin tags and fissures (Crohn's disease)

Rectal examination

The calibre of the anus can be assessed using Hegar's dilators or insertion of a finger. Rectal examination includes palpation of intraluminal faecal masses, assessment of rectal displacement due to intrapelvic masses or fluid collections, and palpation of rectal mucosal lesions (polyps) by sweeping the finger around the rectal wall.

Proctoscopy and sigmoidoscopy

Proctoscopy and sigmoidoscopy are generally performed without bowel preparation. Appropriate sized equipment, a good light source, and suction must be available. Diathermy snare forceps and suction biopsy forceps may be needed to deal with polyps or to obtain mucosa for histology (Fig. 5.44). Following any such procedure, a gauze pack should be left protruding from the anus to act as a wick and to give early warning of bleeding.

Colonoscopy (fibreoptic)

Colonoscopy requires bowel preparation by restricted dietary intake, use of laxatives or enemas, or gut lavage. Though not essential, preoperative in-patient admission may be preferred as a complete colonoscopic examination may take

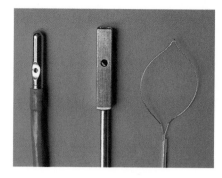

Fig. 5.44 Suction biopsy and diathermy snare forceps available at sigmoidoscopy

a considerable time causing bowel distension and postoperative discomfort. Improved bowel preparation may also be achieved.

Anal dilatation

A gentle digital anal dilatation may help to overcome spasm and pain related to anal fissure and to relieve associated constipation.

Perianal warts

Perianal warts may be too widespread and numerous for medical treatment and require cauterization. The warts may be individually coagulated with diathermy and extensive compound warts may be excised with diathermy. A residual raw surface requires dressing with tullegras. Application of lignocaine gel relieves postoperative discomfort but systemic absorption may occur.

Digital evacuation of faeces

Digital evacuation of faeces may occasionally be necessary in intractable constipation especially in those children with psychological disturbance or whose degree of distress precludes use of enemas and rectal washouts.

Congenital sacrodermal sinus

Congenital sacrodermal sinus is a form of fusion defect and may be associated with a bifid spine. The tract is lined by stratified epithelium and may communicate with the spinal theca. Contamination or infection may result in meningitis and therefore it is recommended that the sinus be excised especially if discharge has ever been noted. Complete communication is not common. The condition should be differentiated from an acquired pilonidal sacrococcygeal sinus or from a coccygeal pit or dimple (Fig. 5.45). Infection should be treated before performing excision.

The child is positioned face down with a sand-bag under the hips to render the sacrum prominent. Lateral traction on the skin of the buttocks by application

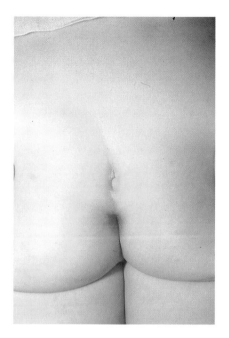

Fig. 5.45 Coccygeal dimple

of adhesive strapping drawn to the edge of the table spreads the natal cleft. Povidone iodine skin cleaning is advisable because of the possibility of faecal contamination.

An elliptical excision is performed around the sinus using a size 11 scalpel blade. The sinus is dissected and the tract isolated and followed to the spinal connection. It is transfixed, ligated, and excised. Haemostasis is achieved and the wound closed primarily with interrupted subcutaneous sutures to obliterate dead space and prevent haematoma formation. The skin is closed with sub-cuticular synthetic absorbable sutures. An occlusive dressing is applied and the parents are advised to keep the area clean and reapply dressings as necessary after passage of stool.

An occasional complication is disruption of the wound. This may follow incomplete closure with haematoma formation or result from pressure or maceration of tissues and sutures due to contamination with faeces or urine. Antibiotic therapy, careful wound cleaning, and re-suturing may be needed.

Tongue-tie

Most cases of tongue-tie are referred because of the parents' worry about speech impediment. Occasionally, a small child may have feeding difficulty or be unable to lick an ice-cream.

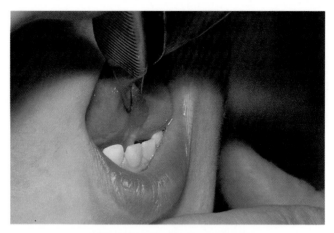

Fig. 5.46 Tongue-tie exposed

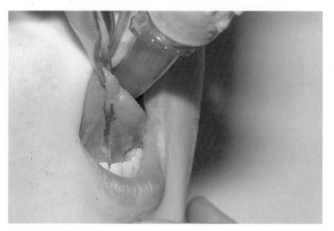

Fig. 5.47 Tongue-tie divided and released

The procedure of division is quick and may be performed without endotracheal intubation by briefly removing the face mask or by using a laryngeal mask. The jaw is held open by the assistant and the tongue tip is grasped by forceps and drawn forward and upwards (Fig. 5.46). The tight frenum (tongue-tie) is divided using fine scissors close to the under surface of the tongue avoiding the frenal artery (Fig. 5.47). It is rarely necessary to ligate a bleeding point unless the artery is inadvertently divided but a 4/0 plain cat gut suture should be available for immediate insertion. The child may drink immediately postoperatively. Infiltration of plain local anaesthetic gives excellent pain relief.

Orthopaedic surgery

Plaster cast application

This is the most common indication for day surgery in paediatric orthopaedics. A general anaesthetic will be required under two circumstances:

(a) to keep the child still so that a limb can be immobilized in a particular position;
(b) when the procedure is expected to be painful.

General anaesthesia will also allow a joint to be examined in more detail either clinically or radiographically. The principal reasons for plaster cast application are congenital dislocation of the hip (CDH) and Perthes' disease. In the former, a hip spica is the usual method of treatment.

Hip spica

Application of a hip spica is shown in Fig. 5.48. Three people are required to apply it safely and well; the person applying the plaster (usually the surgeon), someone to hold the limbs in the correct position, and someone to ensure the safety of the child on the plaster table. The legs are held in around 60° of abduction and just above 90° of flexion at the hip joint. Self-adhesive felt is applied around the abdomen. Plaster wool is then wrapped around both the trunk and the legs. The feet should be included to control rotation. A second roll of wool is wrapped around the abdominal wall to ensure that the cast is not applied too tightly; this is always a possibility when the child is anaesthetized and the respirations are shallow. The plaster is then applied. This may be either plaster of Paris or a synthetic material. If an operation has been performed, a plaster of Paris cast is preferred as it is much easier to remove if necessary. Otherwise, synthetic casting material should be used; it is longer lasting and fewer skin complications are associated with its use. However, when such a cast is applied, great care must be taken to ensure that the edges are smooth and preferably taped. The cast material can be very sharp and a badly applied cast rapidly causes skin sores. When the cast is complete, a bar is applied to strengthen it. It is better positioned posteriorly as this makes carrying the infant easier.

In both Perthes' disease and CDH an added reason for general anaesthesia is that it allows a full examination of the joint. In CDH the question is whether the hip is stable or whether, although it reduces, there is a soft tissue obstruction preventing concentric reduction. An arthrogram is the best and most accurate way of determining this. In Perthes' disease, the examination under anaesthesia may reveal a range of motion quite different from that found in a conscious child. Such an examination is usually supplemented by an arthrogram.

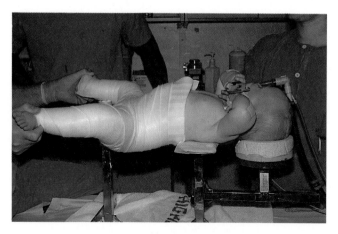

Fig. 5.48   Application of a hip spica

Club foot plaster

A club foot plaster is usually changed under anaesthesia on the first occasion as further manipulation of the foot is then possible. This is inevitably a painful procedure. Subsequent changes without manipulation may be performed in the out-patient clinic.

Arthrogram

An arthrogram may be regarded as an extension of an examination under anaesthesia. Using the image intensifier, it is a dynamic examination. Before the procedure, it must be ascertained that the child has no history of allergy. To minimize the risk of a reaction, a non-ionic radio-opaque contrast medium is recommended. The child is placed on a radiolucent operating table. The skin is prepared and aseptic techniques are used.

The hip joint can be approached from the anterior, lateral, or medial direction. Figure 5.49 shows an antero-lateral approach. The image intensifier is helpful in directing the needle. An 18 gauge needle is adequate for all but the largest children in whom a spinal needle can be used. When the tip of the needle feels as though it is in the joint, an assistant rotates the leg. The femoral head is felt to impinge on the needle tip. A little radio-opaque dye is introduced and a check radiograph is taken. If the needle tip position is satisfactory, further dye is introduced, the needle is removed and the hip moved in all directions to distribute the dye evenly prior to taking further radiographs.

Under radiographic control, the hip is moved around to check the congruency of reduction in the case of CDH or the containment in the case of Perthes'

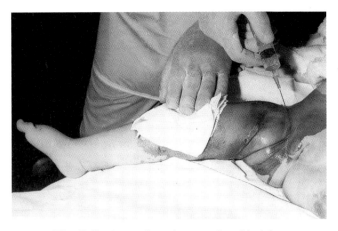

Fig. 5.49 Antero-lateral approach to hip joint

disease. This involves placing the hip first in neutral, then in internal and external rotation, and finally in abduction. The amount of dye seen on the medial side of the femoral head when the hip is in neutral position and then in abduction will show whether the femoral head is adequately reduced. If it is standing off, there will be pooling of dye in the neutral position but this will lessen in abduction. In Perthes' disease, the aim of the examination is to determine whether the femoral head is containable and, if so, in which position. By abducting the hip, the amount of dye medially will show whether hinge abduction is taking place and whether, by performing a varus femoral osteotomy, the hip can be reduced concentrically.

Trigger thumb release

Trigger thumb (or 'snapping thumb') is due to a stenosing tenosynovitis of flexor pollicis longus. Approximately one quarter are bilateral. Clinically, the child has a fixed flexion deformity of up to 60° at the interphalangeal joint (Fig. 5.50). There is a palpable nodule at the base of the thumb just proximal to the metacarpo-phalangeal flexor crease. It moves when the interphalangeal joint is flexed or extended. Attempts to extend the thumb fully or to demonstrate triggering are usually unsuccessful. Many children are first seen in the casualty department with suspected dislocated or fractured thumb and unsuccessful attempts at reduction may have been made.

Trigger thumb is most commonly seen in the first four years of life. Of those that are noted soon after birth, at least 30 per cent recover spontaneously (Dinham and Meggitt 1974) but after the age of six months this figure progressively drops to around 12 per cent by four years old. It is therefore

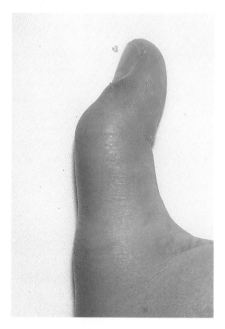

Fig. 5.50 Trigger thumb—flexed interphalangeal joint

reasonable to wait until the child is four to allow spontaneous resolution. Fixed deformities of the interphalangeal joint do not occur up to this time.

Operation

The arm is exsanguinated using an Esmarch bandage and a tourniquet inflated to 100 mm above systolic pressure. Spirit based skin cleansing agents should not be applied as burns may result beneath the tourniquet.

A short transverse incision is made just proximal to the flexor crease at the metacarpo-phalangeal joint (Fig. 5.51). This is usually over the palpable lump. The skin edges are retracted with skin hooks or a small Alm's palpebral retractor. The digital nerves may be seen at the extremes of the incision; dissection proceeds in the midline over the tendon.

The nodule and tendon sheath are exposed. The thumb is flexed and the nodule is palpated. The proximal end of the fibrous flexor sheath is just distal to it. A Watson Cheyne dissector is slipped beneath the sheath which is divided by cutting onto the dissector. The tendon then slides freely and full extension at the interphalangeal joint is possible. A segment of the tendon sheath may be excised to minimize the risk of recurrence. No attempt is made to remove the nodule as it will resolve spontaneously. The wound is closed with a subcuticular suture of nonabsorbable material secured with an adhesive dressing. A cotton wool and crepe bandage is applied for 24 hours. The adhesive dressing and subcuticular suture are removed after one week.

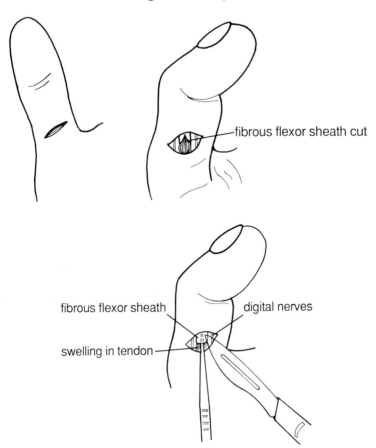

fibrous flexor sheath cut

fibrous flexor sheath

digital nerves

swelling in tendon

Fig. 5.51 Incision for trigger thumb release

Bone cysts and juvenile chronic arthritis

Bone cysts most commonly occur in late childhood (Fig. 5.52a) and may present with a pathological fracture. The results of aspiration and steroid injection of unicameral bone cysts are superior to the alternative of curettage and bone grafting (Oppenheim and Galleno 1984). Two 18 gauge spinal needles with stylets in place are introduced into the cyst under radiographic control. The stylets are removed and straw-coloured fluid aspirated from the cyst confirms the diagnosis. The cyst cavity is irrigated with saline until the fluid return is clear. One needle is then removed and methylprednisolone acetate is instilled: 80–200 mg depending on cyst size is recommended (Campanna *et al.* 1982). The second needle is then removed.

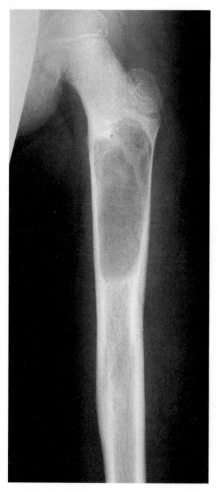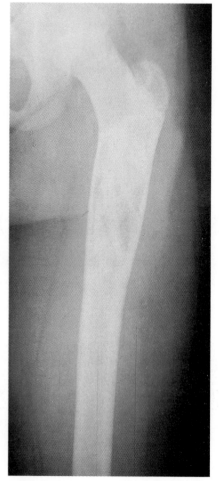

Fig. 5.52a Bone cyst   **Fig. 5.52b** Bone cyst opacified
                                        following aspiration and steroid injection

If there is a danger of pathological fracture (e.g. cyst at proximal femoral
metaphysis) support is advised until healing is under way. When pain has been
a feature, it is often dramatically improved and may have disappeared on
recovery from the anaesthetic. Radiographic follow-up is essential. A satisfactory response is indicated by the cessation of expansion of the cyst and
thickening of the surrounding cortex. The central defect becomes more radio-
opaque (Fig. 5.52*b*), eventually taking on the appearance of frosted glass before
filling in completely. If the response is incomplete, the procedure may be
repeated at intervals of 2−3 months. The results of this simple technique are

gratifying with an overall success rate of 75–95 per cent (Campanna *et al.* 1982; Malawar *et al.* 1985; Smith *et al.* 1985).

Multiple intra articular injections of steroid may be needed in the management of juvenile chronic arthritis.

Arthroscopy

Arthroscopy of the knee joint is occasionally indicated in childhood following acute injuries with positive MRI scan findings. The mobility of the child's knee permits use of the adult sized arthroscope. A tourniquet is routinely used though it does not allow a proper appreciation of the state of the synovium which may be important in suspected juvenile chronic arthritis.

The arthroscope is introduced through an antero-lateral stab incision and the joint space is distended with warm saline. A drain is then introduced into the suprapatellar pouch to allow a through-flow of fluid. Orientation is helped by locating the bubble of air introduced with the fluid which will be on the superior aspect of the joint. Systematic inspection follows:

(1) back of patella;
(2) femoral condyles;
(3) menisci;
(4) tibial plateau and condyles;
(5) cruciate ligaments.

Lesions such as discoid menisci, loose bodies, and osteochondritis dissecans are noted. A hook introduced through a separate stab incision may be used to lift and examine menisci and articular cartilage.

At conclusion of the examination the joint is irrigated and the puncture wounds are closed with interrupted sutures or adhesive strips. A cotton wool and crepe bandage is applied and the patient is allowed to walk immediately within the limits of comfort.

Minor toe surgery

Flexor tenotomy

This is indicated for symptomatic curly toe. Whether it will respond to a flexor tenotomy can be simply assessed (Fig. 5.53). The affected toe is held with the metatarsal phalangeal (MTP) joint in flexion and extension of the inter-phalangeal (IP) joint is attempted. It is usually possible without much difficulty. The MTP joint is then extended. This puts tension onto the sublimis tendon and, if it is tight, the IP joint will not be able to be maintained in extension. In such a case, flexor tenotomy will be helpful.

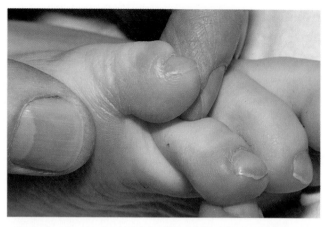

Fig. 5.53a Curly fourth toe—in straight position with metacarpophalangeal joint flexed and interphalangeal joint extended

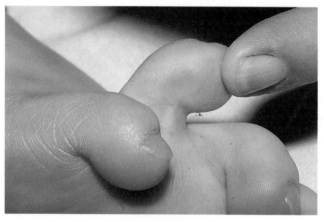

Fig. 5.53b Curly fourth toe—becomes flexed when metacarpophalangeal joint is extended

The procedure is performed with the patient supine. The leg is exsanguinated using an Esmarch bandage and a tourniquet is applied to the upper thigh at a pressure about 100 mm above systolic blood pressure. The incision is made on the dorsal lateral aspect of the toe obliquely just distal to the MTP joint (Fig. 5.54). Mosquito forceps are used to spread the soft tissues. The neurovascular bundle is just below this on the plantar aspect of the wound. The tip of the forceps is advanced to the plantar surface of the proximal phalanx. The fibrous flexor sheath is found at this point. It is incised longitudinally for 1 cm so that the tip of the forceps can be introduced across the sheath. The forceps

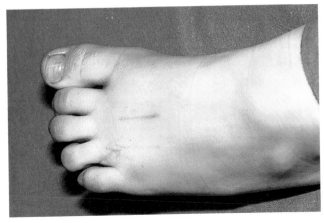

Fig. 5.54 Incision for extensor tenotomy of toe

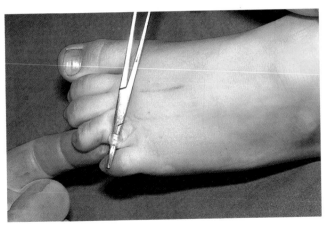

Fig. 5.55 Flexor tendon hooked out by forceps prior to division to release curly toe

are used to hook out the flexor tendon (Fig. 5.55) which is then divided. The toe may not immediately extend fully and manipulation into hyperextension may be required. Bupivacaine is instilled into the wound which is closed with a subcuticular suture. A cotton wool and crepe bandage is applied for 24 hours.

Removal of a nail

A Jacques catheter is applied around the base of the digit as a tourniquet after elevation of the limb for one minute. A sharp pointed pair of scissors is introduced under the nail and pushed down beneath the lunula. The ends are spread to detach the nail from its bed. Kocher forceps are used to avulse the nail. The raw nail bed is dressed with a non-adherent soft paraffin gauze dressing and a crepe bandage is applied. This will need to be soaked off at the first dressing change. Dressings are continued for 10 days.

Nail bed ablation

The nail is first removed as above. Incisions are then made at each corner of the base of the nail and flaps lifted. The surrounding skin is smeared with soft paraffin to protect it from 50% phenol which is applied to the corners of the nail bed for one minute using an orange stick. Dressings are applied as for simple nail removal.

Specialized scans

General anaesthesia and day stay may be required for isotope, CT, and MRI scans for:

(1) staging of tumours;
(2) assessment of the anatomy of congenital malformations (e.g. club foot, proximal focal femoral deficiency);
(3) preoperative planning (e.g. complex congenital dislocation of the hip requiring 3-dimensional reconstruction of the joint).

Excision of ganglion

These small cystic swellings associated with joints or tendons contain gelatinous fluid and may ramify into surrounding tissues. Many disappear spontaneously but others may be tender, ache, or appear unsightly. Careful excision through a skin crease incision is best performed with exsanguination and tourniquet.

Removal of fixation devices

Protruding pins and external fixation devices may be easily removed with local or no anaesthesia. However, in the young or frightened child or when the procedure involves significant discomfort, general anaesthesia may be needed.

Ophthalmic surgery

At present, intra-ocular surgery in children requires hospital admission, but most procedures in ophthalmic surgery which do not involve opening the eye itself may be carried out as day cases. There is a long tradition of non-surgical day case procedures in paediatric ophthalmology including:

(1) EUA combined with refraction;
(2) intra-ocular pressure measurement;
(3) ultrasonography;
(4) electrophysiology.

Anaesthetic techniques such as intramuscular or intravenous Ketamine are necessary for intra-ocular pressure measurement.

Probing of tear passages

Probing of the tear passages is now less commonly performed due to an increasing awareness of the tendency for congenital nasolacrimal duct obstruction to resolve spontaneously. As a consequence of this change in practice, children with persistent epiphora may well have 'high-level' block with canalicular or punctal pathology and the genuine cases of nasolacrimal duct obstruction are older. Therefore, examination of the upper tear passages is important. If they are normal, then it is customary to pass a standard lacrimal probe via the upper punctum into the tear sac, down the duct, and into the nose (Fig. 5.56). The probe is passed posteriorly and medially but considerable doubt exists as to how often the probe goes accurately down the duct. Studies with contrast medium show a high incidence of false passage. Despite this, the procedure has a high success rate. Patency can be checked by testing for the presence of the probe in the nose or by syringing the passages with air or saline.

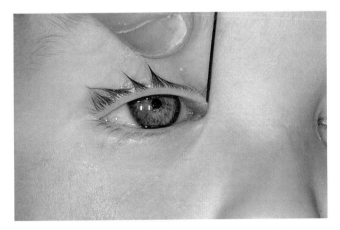

Fig. 5.56 Lacrimal probe passed down tear duct

Chalazion

Cysts of the eyelid (chalazion) are common in children and may require surgery because they are large, multiple, or bilateral. A chalazion clamp is used and a radial incision is made in the conjunctiva over the centre of the cyst after eversion of the eyelid (Fig. 5.57). Bleeding must be controlled during the procedure to allow accuracy. Following curettage of the cyst contents and removal of the clamp, bleeding is usually profuse although short-lived. An eyepad is applied and retained in place for 20 minutes to control oozing. It is then removed. The child is encouraged to bathe the eye and to use topical antibiotic drops 6 hourly for 3 days.

Tarsorrhaphy

Tarsorrhaphy is helpful in two situations:

(1) recurrent epithelial breakdown due to congenital trigeminal anaesthesia;
(2) redundant lax lids (euryblepharon).

Lateral tarsorrhaphy is used. As it is permanent, the posterior lid margin as well as an intermarginal strip is removed. Two double-armed 5/0 silk sutures are passed through the split lids and tied over bolsters (e.g. rubber) (Fig. 5.58). Antibiotic drops are instilled 6 hourly for 3 days and the sutures are removed after 14 days.

Conjunctival cyst/stitch granuloma

These are rare complications of squint surgery (Fig. 5.59). The best approach to obtain good exposure and minimal bleeding is through the original incision. An operating microscope may be needed for complete dissection of the implantation conjunctival cyst or complete removal of suture material or granulation tissue.

Squint surgery

An up-to-date assessment of orthoptic status is needed immediately prior to surgery for squint. All squints are suitable for day case surgery. A limbal incision is usually made and absorbable sutures (e.g. 5/0 Vicryl) are used. Rectus recession is performed using a 'hang-back' technique. The parents should be warned in advance about the operative bruising expected following inferior oblique muscle recession.

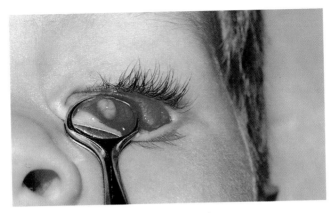

Fig. 5.57 Chalazion

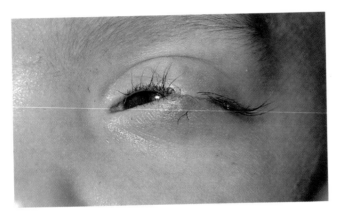

Fig. 5.58 Tarsorrhaphy

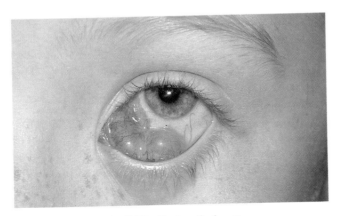

Fig. 5.59 Conjunctival cyst

Other extra-ocular ophthalmic procedures

Although other extra-ocular ophthalmic procedures may be suitable for day case surgery, continuing concern regarding complications limits changes in the standard practice of in-patient surgery. Examples are:

(1) ptosis surgery—risk of breaching corneal integrity and of postoperative infection;
(2) dacryocystorhinostomy—risk of postoperative bleeding.

Dental surgery

General anaesthesia as an aid to providing dental care has a long history; Napoleon III had a tooth extracted in front of admiring courtiers following the administration of nitrous oxide. Recently, a report from the Department of Health (1990) highlighted the need for adequate facilities for dental surgery under general anaesthesia and drew up a list of recommendations. These are better met by a hospital day bed unit than by a dental surgery. It is possible to perform most types of dental treatment under general anaesthesia on a day case basis. The limiting factors are associated medical conditions (congenital heart disease, diabetes, renal failure) and the time taken for some procedures. For general anaesthesia, a laryngeal mask is most suitable; its only disadvantage is the larger size compared with an endotracheal tube. Recently a new design of laryngeal mask airway with a narrower reinforced non-kinking tube has become available which is useful for dental work (Haynes and Morton 1993). In a recent study fewer desaturation episodes due to airway problems were noted in paediatric out-patient dental patients managed with a laryngeal mask, compared with a similar group in whom a nasal mask was used (Baillie et al. 1991).

A gauze or sponge pack is inserted around the tube to seal the pharynx and collect debris and fragments. Treatment is usually performed with the patient lying horizontal and the head supported in a ring to reduce movement.

The equipment used for day case dental treatment includes a mobile dental cart fitted with high and low speed dental drills and air/water spray syringe. It is powered by a 7 bar compressed air supply and carries a self-contained sterile water system. The unit is also fitted with one-way valves to prevent aspiration of contaminated water into the system. The handpieces and air/water syringe are autoclavable. The whole unit is designed to be readily cleaned after each case. A mobile drawer unit holds dental materials and the supply of sterile packed dental instruments. An automatic mixer and visible light curing unit are also used.

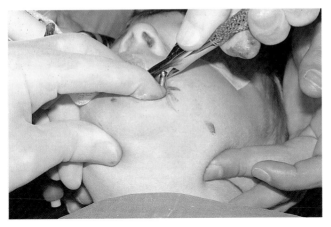

Fig. 5.60 Support of the mandible is required for extraction of lower teeth even when a laryngeal mask is used

Dental procedures performed under general anaesthesia as day cases are:

1. Extractions: extractions may be necessary both on account of caries and for orthodontic reasons. Additional head support is needed for extractions to counteract the force of the extraction procedures and to protect the airway. This is especially important during extraction of lower teeth (Fig. 5.60). For the extraction of a small number of primary teeth, the laryngeal mask may be dispensed with and the teeth extracted using a nasal mask and a suitable throat pack to protect the airway.
2. Restorations: both posterior and anterior restorations are carried out using various types of dental material. Root canal therapy is also performed.
3. Periodontal treatment: periodontal treatment includes scaling to remove plaque and calculus.
4. Biopsies and minor oral surgery: procedures such as excision of mucous retention cysts.
5. Fissure sealants: following etching of the occlusal surface of the posterior teeth, a plastic resin coating is used to seal the grooves and prevent caries.

ENT procedures

Provision of a binocular operating microscope is necessary specifically for use in a day case ENT theatre. Transfer of delicate optical equipment between theatres leads rapidly to degradation of performance. A variety of more minor ear, nose, throat, and laryngotracheobronchial procedures with a low incidence of postoperative risk are possible on a day case basis.

Ear operations and investigations

In view of the tendency of serous *otitis media* to resolve spontaneously, it is important that age-appropriate audiological testing and tympanometry is available immediately prior to surgery. The commonest procedures performed are myringotomy with or without grommet insertion, examination of the ears under anaesthesia, and suction clearance. Other procedures are:

(a) brain stem auditory evoked response audiometry which may be indicated when there is difficulty in establishing auditory thresholds by co-operative methods. General anaesthesia may be preferable to sedation as it is more predictable and has minimal effect on response levels;
(b) electrocochleography;
(c) myringoplasty and tympanoplasty;
(d) removal of foreign body.

Nasal operations and procedures

(a) manipulation of fractured nasal bones;
(b) removal of foreign body from the nasal cavity;
(c) submucosal diathermy of the inferior turbinates;
(d) antral wash-out;
(e) sinoscopy.

Laryngotracheobronchial procedures

Laryngotracheobronchial examination requires close monitoring in the post-operative period as a small degree of oedema may lead to obstruction. In-patient admission is usually indicated postoperatively but, when repeated procedures of the same type have been performed with consistently good postoperative progress, day case surgery may be considered in the individual case. Laser vaporization of laryngeal papillomata may be performed as a day case procedure on this basis.

Tonsillectomy and adenoidectomy

Although some studies have suggested that day case tonsillectomy is a safe procedure when carried out on carefully selected patients, there is general concern that the level of postoperative risk remains too high. Specific criteria for exclusion are:

(a) age under 36 months;
(b) evidence of sleep apnoea.

The principal complications of tonsillectomy with or without adenoidectomy are:

1. Primary haemorrhage. Primary haemorrhage occurs in up to 0.5 per cent of cases usually within the first 12 hours after surgery (Capper and Randall 1984). Careful postoperative monitoring is necessary to detect changes in vital signs suggesting blood loss but the first evidence of primary haemorrhage may be vomiting of large quantities of altered blood. A further general anaesthetic may be necessary to allow identification and control of the source of bleeding.

2. Dehydration. Dehydration may occur due to inadequate fluid intake postoperatively as a result of apprehension or pain. Oral fluid replacement with monitoring to ensure adequate intake may be sufficient but, in some cases, intravenous fluid replacement may be required. The extent of pre-operative fasting must be taken into account when assessing requirements. Inadequate fluid therapy and hydration may increase the incidence of secondary haemorrhage due to infection.

3. Inadequate control of pain. The pain of the tonsillectomy procedure may require paracetamol (oral), diclofenac sodium (suppository), or opiates (intramuscular or intravenous) for adequate control; the latter is, in itself, an indication for in-patient admission.

4. Postoperative vomiting.

These potential postoperative complications following tonsillectomy and adenoidectomy cause considerable concern in relation to day surgery and careful audit of changes from the traditional pattern of 24–48 hour hospital admission is required for these procedures.

References

Baillie, R., Barnett, M. B., and Fraser, J. F. (1991). The brain laryngeal mask: a comparative study with the nasal mask in paediatric dental outpatient anaesthesia. *Anaesthesia*, **46**, 358–60.

Campanna, R., Dalmonte, A., Gitelis, S., *et al.* (1982). The natural history of unilateral bone cyst after steroid injection. *Clinical Orthopaedics and Related Research*, **166**, 209–11.

Capper, J. W. R. and Randall, C. (1984). Post-operative haemorrhage in tonsillectomy and adenoidectomy in children. *Journal of Laryngology and Otology*, **98**, 363–5.

Cooper, G. G., Thomson, G. J. L., and Raine, P. A. M. (1983). Therapeutic retraction of the foreskin in childhood. *British Medical Journal*, **286**, 186–7.

Dinham, J. M. and Meggitt, B. F. (1974). Trigger thumbs in children. *Journal of Bone and Joint Surgery*, **56B**, 153–5.

Fyfe, A. H. B. and Azmy, A. (1992). Personal communication.

Gordon, A. and Collin, J. (1993). Save the normal foreskin. *British Medical Journal*, **306**, 1–2.

108 Surgical techniques

Gyrtrup, J. H. K., Mejdahl, S., *et al.* (1989). Outpatient orchidopexy and herniotomy in children. *Acta Paediatrica Scandinavica*, **78**, 754–8.

Haynes, S. R. and Morton, N. S. (1993). The laryngeal mask airway: a review of its use in paediatric anaesthesia. *Paediatric Anaesthesia*, **3**, 65–73.

John Radcliffe Hospital Cryptorchidism Study Group (1986). Cryptorchidism: an apparent substantial increase since 1960. *British Medical Journal*, **293**, 1401–4.

Langer, J. C., Chandling, B., and Rosenberg, M. (1987). Intraoperative bupivacaine during outpatient hernia repair in children; a randomised double blind trial. *Journal of Paediatric Surgery*, **22**, 267–70.

Malawar *et al.* (abstract) (1985). Unilateral bone cysts treated by renografin injection and intracavity methylprednisolone acetate. *Journal of Pediatric Orthopedics*, **5**, 499.

Mejdahl, S. and Gyrtrup, J. H. K. (1989). Outpatient operation of inguinal hernia in children. *British Journal of Surgery*, **76**, 406–7.

Melone, J. H., Schwartz, M. Z., Tyson, K. R. T., *et al.* (1992). Outpatient inguinal herniorrhaphy in premature infants; is it safe? *Journal of Pediatric Surgery*, **27**, 203–8.

Moir, C. R., Blair, G. K., Fraser, G. C. *et al.*, (1987). The emerging pattern of pediatric day-care surgery. *Journal of Pediatric Surgery*, **22**, 743–5.

Moores, M. A., Wandless, J. G., and Fell, D. (1990). Paediatric postoperative analgesia; a comparison of rectal diclofenac with caudal bupivacaine after inguinal herniotomy. *Anaesthesia*, **45**, 156–8.

NHS in Scotland, Management Executive (1992). A guide to consent to examination, investigation, treatment or operation.

O'Donnell, B. and Puri, P. (1984). Treatment of vesico-ureteric reflux by endoscopic injection of Teflon. *British Medical Journal*, **289**, 7–9.

Oppenheim, L. and Galleno, H. (1984). Operative treatment versus steroid injection in the management of unicameral bone cysts. *Journal of Pediatric Orthopedics*, **4**, 1–7.

Smith, *et al.* (abstract) (1985). Early results of steroid injections in unilateral bone cysts. *Journal of Pediatric Orthopaedics*, **5**, 499.

Williams, N., Chel, J., and Kapila, L. (1993). Why are children referred for circumcision. *British Medical Journal*, **306**, 28.

Yang, C. D. (1991). (Day care surgery of inguinal hernia and hydrocele of children.) *Chung-Hua-Wai-Ko-Tsa-Chih*, **29**, 278–80.

6 Postoperative management

RECOVERY FROM ANAESTHESIA
N. S. Morton

Immediate recovery from anaesthesia and surgery should be in a fully equipped recovery area with a one-to-one ratio of personnel trained in paediatric nursing. Pulse oximetry, facilities for oxygen therapy, and suction equipment must be provided. A tilting trolley with suitably padded sides is ideal for nursing the child in this area. Monitoring of vital signs, adequacy of protective airway reflexes, and correct positioning to prevent airway obstruction, regurgitation, and aspiration are the priorities. The nurse also monitors the wound site for bleeding, checks the security of dressings, and the adequacy of pain relief.

Recovery is usually swift and uncomplicated, particularly if the principles of balanced anaesthesia and analgesia noted above are followed. The main factors influencing the rate of recovery include the use of premedicant drugs, the induction and maintenance techniques, the analgesic techniques, the age of the patient, and the duration of the surgery.

The majority of paediatric day cases do not require premedication but when required, midazolam (orally or intranasally), ketamine (intramuscularly), or methohexitone (rectally) do not significantly prolong recovery.

Inhalational induction and maintenance produce the most rapid recovery. In comparative trials of the currently used agents, enflurane comes out best in terms of rate of recovery (Simmons et al. 1989; Lerman 1992). Sevoflurane induction and maintenance results in more rapid recovery than halothane induction and maintenance in children (Naito et al. 1991). Desflurane induction and maintenance produces particularly rapid recovery (Taylor and Lerman 1992; Zwass et al. 1992). To gain the advantages of halothane during induction and more rapid awakening, it has been suggested that after halothane induction, maintenance should be with isoflurane (Pandit et al. 1985).

Recovery after propofol induction is quicker than after thiopentone induction, when a volatile agent is used for maintenance (Runcie et al. 1993). This is not the case for more prolonged procedures. Pain is a confounding variable in many studies of recovery and may explain the small differences found in some studies comparing recovery after IV induction. There is a need for standardization of the operation, regional block, and other analgesics to give more valid comparisons. The child in severe pain will awaken sooner than the pain free child.

Recently, propofol induction and maintenance was compared with propofol induction/halothane maintenance in children who had had regional blocks and no difference in recovery could be demonstrated (Doyle *et al.* 1993). In another study, after halothane induction, propofol infusion maintenance produced quicker recovery than halothane maintenance (Watcha *et al.* 1991). A potential disadvantage of very rapid awakening and rapid surgery, is that the regional block may not have become fully effective by the time the child is recovering. This is especially true for blocks performed using bupivacaine which may take up to 15 minutes to achieve its full effect. It is not unusual in the author's hospital for operations such as herniotomy and circumcision to last much less than 15 minutes.

Assessment of recovery to predetermined milestones such as eye opening or giving name correctly, are more sensitive than assessments of fitness for discharge, such as the Steward scoring system (Puttick and Rosen 1988; Steward 1975) when comparing the influence of anaesthetic techniques on recovery. However, the Steward score is a useful basis for defining discharge criteria (vide infra).

Parental involvement in the early recovery phase is encouraged in many units (McConachie *et al.* 1989). We favour parental involvement with the conscious child on return from the recovery area to the day ward. The presence of the parent affords reassurance and comfort and is effective in reducing postoperative distress and anxiety and the requirement for sedation. However, the parent must be prepared for this role and will need reassurance and information about the degree of distress to be expected, the possibility of some blood staining (e.g. tongue-tie release), and how best to position or hold the child.

In the recovery area, the parent will need to be supervised by a nurse who should be prepared for the possibilities of the parent becoming distressed or fainting or the parent taking inappropriate action with the child. A combination of tact and firmness is necessary in this supporting role.

POSTOPERATIVE CARE

P. A. M. Raine, C. J. Best and D. J. M. Fretwell

Postoperative feeding

As soon as the child has recovered consciousness, he may be offered a drink or light snack in most cases. However, exceptions should be made following endotracheal intubation and some dental or oral procedures. As the parents may have fasted preoperatively with the child, they may also be in need of sustenance.

Postoperative 'ward round'

At the conclusion of the session, the surgeon, anaesthetist, and nurse will wish to review the patients before discharge in order to:

1. discuss the procedure with the parents;
2. check suitability for discharge;
3. explain the postoperative plans and arrangements for review; and
4. answer questions and anxieties.

The presence of the liaison district nurse is valuable in allowing arrangements to be followed through and providing an additional point of contact for the parent.

Postoperative instructions

In addition to discussion with the parents, written postoperative instructions should be issued in order to reinforce information such as:

1. simple explanation of the procedure;
2. the type of incision and dressing;
3. the nature of sutures and the need for suture removal;
4. the measures to be taken to control postoperative pain;
5. when to resume normal diet;
6. restrictions on postoperative activity;
7. when to allow bathing or washing;
8. notes on special care of the wound and problems which should be reported, e.g. redness, swelling, discharge, or unpleasant odour;
9. what to do if problems arise—contact names and telephone number for the hospital or general practitioner should be given;
10. arrangements for follow-up by the district nurse or general practitioner;
11. arrangements for review at the hospital out-patient clinic.

DISCHARGE CRITERIA

N. S. Morton

The Steward score (Steward 1975), assesses the safe return of protective reflexes. Wakefulness, ventilation, and movement are tested and are assigned a score of 0, 1, or 2. However, discharge criteria should be broader in scope

Table 6.1 Discharge criteria

1. Vital signs normal for age.
2. Conscious level normal.
3. Protective airway reflexes fully regained (swallowing, coughing, gag reflexes).
4. No respiratory distress.
5. No stridor.
6. Appropriate movement.
7. No nausea and vomiting.
8. Able to drink and tolerate clear fluids.
9. No bleeding.
10. No unexpected intraoperative events.
11. Escorted home by responsible parent/guardian.
12. Private or taxi transport provided.
13. Full written and verbal instructions concerning postoperative care given.
14. Clear instructions given concerning line of contact for parent/guardian in the event of problems.

to take account of age, preoperative assessment, surgical, and social factors (Table 6.1). Vital signs should be normal for the child's age. there should be no respiratory distress or stridor, particularly in those children who have been intubated. The conscious level should be normal for the child's age and pre-operative condition (e.g. mentally handicapped child). Protective airway reflexes should be fully regained and this would include swallowing, coughing, and gag reflexes. The child should be able to move appropriately for his age. Motor blockade secondary to caudal epidural blockade or as a complication of inguinal block may preclude discharge in older, normally ambulant children but is less important in the small infant.

Nausea and vomiting should be unusual in modern practice, but may preclude discharge. Emesis can be particularly troublesome after squint surgery, orchidopexy, and gastroscopy. It can be minimized

(a) by the use of propofol for induction and/or maintenance (Watcha *et al.* 1991) (because of its anti-emetic effects);
(b) use of local anaesthesia rather than opioids for pain relief; and
(c) avoidance of endotracheal intubation.

In our practice, for example, the incidence of emesis after squint surgery is less than 10 per cent when a technique comprising propofol induction, spontaneous breathing via a laryngeal mask airway, diclofenac and amethocaine eye drops is used (personal observations). New anti-emetics such as ondansetron may have a role in day case surgery. It has a superior safety profile in children compared with agents such as metoclopramide, which have a high incidence of extra-pyramidal side effects. Ability to drink and tolerate clear fluids is desirable, but adequately hydrated children can be discharged prior to drinking if they meet the other discharge criteria.

Bleeding may necessitate re-operation and/or in-patient admission for observation. Pain may require the use of opioids on an in-patient basis. The surgical procedure may unexpectedly become more extensive or prolonged and justify in-patient postoperative care.

Any unexpected intraoperative events such as regurgitation, aspiration, bronchospasm, hypersensitivity reactions, suxamethonium apnoea, or suspected malignant hyperpyrexia warrant admission for further investigation and treatment. Post-extubation stridor requires careful observation and treatment in an intensive care area.

Reasons for hospital admission

It follows from the above that a small number of children will require overnight admission for one of a number of reasons. This contingency should be considered at the time of planning a day admission and the parent should be aware of the possibility and have considered how best to deal with the enforced change of plan. The reasons for admission are:

1. persistently abnormal vital signs or conscious level;
2. any suggestion of a problem with the airway;
3. motor blockade;
4. persistent nausea and vomiting;
5. haemorrhage;
6. severe pain;
7. a longer than expected surgical procedure;
8. hypotension and faintness;
9. difficulty with the surgical procedure requiring more extensive dissection and 'surgical trauma';
10. postoperative wound problem, e.g. separation;
11. for care after unexpected intraoperative events.

In centres with well-established day care programmes the hospital in-patient admission rate has been between 1 and 2 per cent (Moir et al. 1987; Postuma et al. 1987).

FOLLOW-UP AND AUDIT
P. A. M. Raine and D. J. M. Fretwell

Discharge letter

An immediate discharge letter should be completed and sent directly to the GP on the day of the procedure or given to the parent for delivery. The letter will contain details of the diagnosis, procedure, special requirements, arrangements for follow-up, and a contact in case of unforeseen need.

Transport home

All paediatric day cases must be escorted home by a responsible parent or guardian. The child should be transported home by car or taxi preferably accompanied by another adult in addition to the driver. In instances where this has not been satisfactorily planned prior to the day admission, arrangements to transport the child home by ambulance or for overnight admission may be required. The child should not be allowed to travel home on public transport.

Postoperative home visit

The paediatric trained district nurse has a special and important role in the proper functioning of a day care surgical programme (Atwell and Gow 1985). Ideally, all children will be seen at home postoperatively but in many cases it is practical to offer this service only to those patients whose needs have been identified prior to or at the time of the admission. The district nurse will be involved in: postoperative wound care, removal of dressings, removal of sutures, reinforcement and reiteration of advice to parents, assessment and provision of pain relief, and support and advice for parents.

Not all day case surgical patients will require further hospital out-patient review and this may be restricted to procedures such as cosmetic surgery (e.g. minor cleft lip revision), orchidopexy, and hypospadias repair. However, such appointments offer the opportunity to audit not only the outcome of the surgical procedure but also the outcome for the child and family of day case as opposed to in-patient admission (Campbell *et al.* 1988). Such audit is essential if the benefits of day case surgery are to continue to outweigh the possible risks of earlier discharge and if the scope and spectrum of day case surgery are to widen in a properly controlled manner.

References

Atwell, J. D. and Gow, M. A. (1985). Paediatric trained district nurse in the community; expensive luxury or economic necessity? *British Medical Journal*, **291**, 227–9.

Campbell, I. R., Scaife, J. M., and Johnstone, J. M. (1988). Psychological effects of day case surgery compared with inpatient surgery. *Archives of Disease in Childhood*, **63**, 415–7.

Doyle, E., McFadzean, W., and Morton, N. S. (1993). I.V. anaesthesia with propofol using a target-controlled infusion system: comparison with inhalation anaesthesia for general surgical procedures in children. *British Journal of Anaesthesia*, **70**, 542–5.

Lerman, J. (1992). Pharmacology of inhalational anesthetics in infants and children. *Paediatric Anaesthesia*, **2**, 191–203.

McConachie, I. W., Day, A., and Morris, P. (1989). Recovery from anaesthesia in children. *Anaesthesia*, **44**, 986–90.

Naito, Y., Tamai, S., Shingu, K., Fujimori, R., and Mori, K. (1991). Comparison between sevoflurane and halothane for paediatric ambulatory anaesthesia. *British Journal of Anaesthesia*, **67**, 387–9.

Pandit, U. A., Stende, G. M., and Leach, A. B. (1985). Induction and recovery characteristics of isoflurane and halothane anaesthesia for short outpatient procedures in children. *Anaesthesia*, **40**, 1226–30.

Postuma, R. R., Ferguson, C. C., Stanwick, R. S., *et al.* (1987). Pediatric day-care surgery: a 30 year hospital experience. *Journal of Pediatric Surgery*, **22**, 304–7.

Puttick, N. and Rosen, M. (1988). Propofol induction and maintenance with nitrous oxide in paediatric outpatient dental anaesthesia. *Anaesthesia*, **43**, 646–9.

Runcie, C. J., MacKenzie, S., Arthur, D. S., and Morton, N. S. (1993). Comparison of recovery from anaesthesia induced in children with either propofol or thiopentone. *British Journal of Anaesthesia*, **70**, 192–5.

Simmons, M., Miller, C. D., Cummings, G. C., and Todd, J. G. (1989). Outpatient paediatric dental anaesthesia. A comparison of halothane, enflurane and isoflurane. *Anaesthesia*, **44**, 735–8.

Steward, D. J. (1975). A simplified scoring system for the postoperative recovery room. *Canadian Anaesthetists' Society Journal*, **22**, 111–13.

Taylor, R. and Lerman, J. (1992). Induction and recovery characteristics of desflurane in infants and children. *Canadian Journal of Anaesthesia*, **39**, 6–13.

Watcha, M. F., Simeon, R. M., White, P. F., and Stevens, J. L. (1991). Effect of propofol on the incidence of postoperative vomiting after strabismus surgery in pediatric outpatients. *Anesthesiology*, **75**, 204–9.

Zwass, M. S., Fisher, D. M., Welborn, L. G., Coté, C. J., Davis, P. J., Dinner, M., *et al.* (1992). Induction and maintenance characteristics of anaesthesia with desflurane and nitrous oxide in infants and children. *Anesthesiology*, **76**, 373–8.

Index